AMERICAN JOURNAL of PUBLIC HEALTH
JULY 2024
Issue 7

AJPH

A PUBLICATION OF THE
AMERICAN PUBLIC HEALTH ASSOCIATION

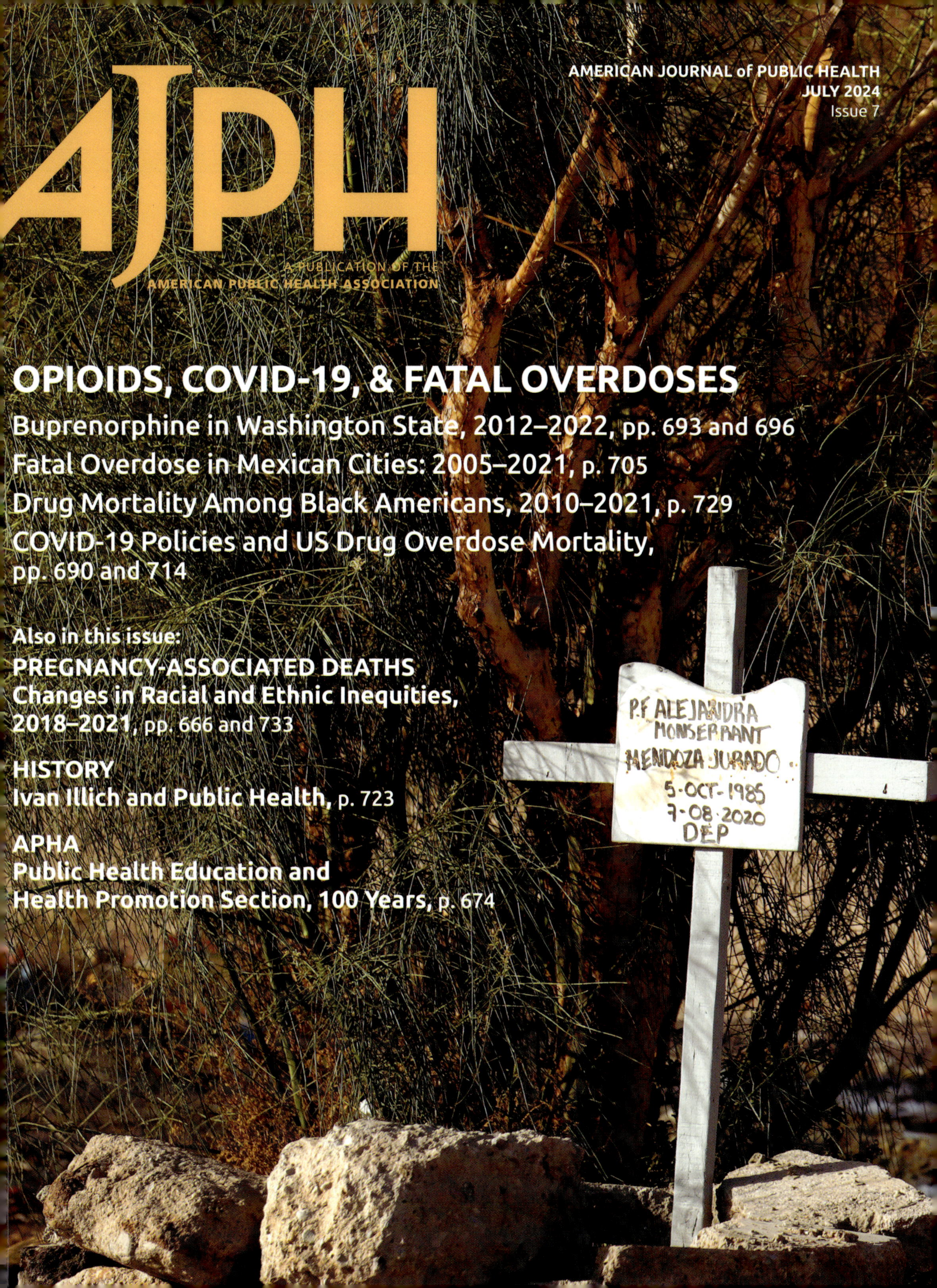

OPIOIDS, COVID-19, & FATAL OVERDOSES

Buprenorphine in Washington State, 2012–2022, pp. 693 and 696

Fatal Overdose in Mexican Cities: 2005–2021, p. 705

Drug Mortality Among Black Americans, 2010–2021, p. 729

COVID-19 Policies and US Drug Overdose Mortality, pp. 690 and 714

Also in this issue:

PREGNANCY-ASSOCIATED DEATHS
Changes in Racial and Ethnic Inequities, 2018–2021, pp. 666 and 733

HISTORY
Ivan Illich and Public Health, p. 723

APHA
Public Health Education and Health Promotion Section, 100 Years, p. 674

AJPH®, published monthly, is the official Journal of the American Public Health Association®, 800 I St NW, Washington, DC 20001-3710; (202) 777- APHA; TDD (202) 777-2500. APHA is a nongovernmental professional society founded in 1872, representing all disciplines and specialties in public health.

The *American Journal of Public Health*® (*AJPH*) (print ISSN: 0090-0036; electronic ISSN: 1541- 0048), first published in 1911, is the official journal of the American Public Health Association® (APHA). The oldest and largest organization of public health professionals in the world, APHA represents approximately 30 000 members from more than 50 occupations of public health.

Submissions: Visit www.editorialmanager.com/ajph or ajph.edmgr.com for online manuscript preparation and submission guidelines. Contributions of original unpublished research, social science analyses, scholarly essays, critical commentaries, departments, and letters to the editor are welcome. Questions? Write ajph.submissions@apha.org or call APHA at (202) 777-2469.

Print plus online subscriptions: Institutional price (print copy with online access for a single institution and all authorized users, regardless of geographic location) varies by size of organization and ranges from $993–$1445 for US organizations, and $1073–$1526 for international organizations (air delivery); multiple campuses not permitted without special arrangement. Details of the tiered pricing system at https://subscriptionoffice.com/pages/apha-landing-page. To order, write apha.subscriptions@apha.org.

Online-only subscriptions: Institutional price for one institution and its authorized users (regardless of geographic location) is $878–$1307. To order, write apha.subscriptions@apha.org. For academic consortia or multisite corporate subscriptions, contact apha.subscriptions@apha.org.

Print-only subscriptions: Institutional price is US $701, $782 international.

Back print issues: A limited number of print issues are for sale. Single copies are US $49, $55 international (air delivery). Shipping included; prepay only. To order, write apha.subscriptions@apha.org.

Reprints: For prices and ordering information on 50 or more reprints, check the Reprints section at www.ajph.org. To order smaller quantities of reprints (rush delivery), use the "Purchase Article" link on the article site itself.

Electronic access: Online articles more than 10 years old are available free for personal use at www.ajph.org. Recent articles are available through pay-per-view: single PDF article for $24, single issue access for 24 hours for $33, or entire site access for 24 hours for $38.

Postal information: Periodicals postage paid at Washington, DC, and additional mailing offices. Postmaster: Send address changes to American Journal of Public Health, 800 I St NW, Washington, DC 20001-3710.

Address changes: Send to AJPH, Membership Department (members) or AJPH Subscriptions (subscribers), APHA, 800 I St NW, Washington, DC 20001-3710. Or write to membership.mail@apha. org (members) or apha.subscriptions@apha.org (subscribers).

Advertising: For pricing and other information, see www.ajph.org. Please write to ashell.alston@apha.org or call (202) 777-2470 for other advertising opportunities. Ask about special exhibit packages and sponsorships. Acceptance of advertising by the *Journal* does not imply endorsement of products.

Indexes: Publications that index or abstract articles from AJPH include the following: Ageline, Assia (Applied Social Science Index and Abstracts), Biological Abstracts, Chemical Abstracts, CINAHL, Criminal Justice Abstracts, EMBASE, EMCare, Environmental Abstracts, e-psyche, ERIC, ETOH (Alcohol and Alcohol Problems Science Database), Excerpta Medica, Food Science and Technology, General Science Index, Grateful Med, Hospital Literature Index, Human Resources Abstracts, International Pharmaceutical Abstracts (IPA), Medline, Physical Education Index, Pollution Abstracts, Psychological Abstracts, PsychINFO, Safety Science Abstracts, Sage Family Studies Abstracts, Sage Human Resources Abstracts, Science Citation Index, SCOPUS, SIIC Data Bases, Social Work Research and Abstracts, and Statistical Reference Index (SRI)/LexisNexis.

AJPH

A PUBLICATION OF THE
AMERICAN PUBLIC HEALTH ASSOCIATION

COVER: Mexicali, Mexico, June 7, 2023. A cross was put up for Alejandra Monserrante Mendoza Jurado, who died of an overdose on August 7, 2020. She lived with other homeless people in an empty lot, where they do drugs in Mexicali. Most all of the heroin and meth drugs in Mexicali have traces of fentanyl, leading to a high death rate among addicts. Even if they wanted to avoid fentanyl, it would be impossible.

Cover concept and image selection by Aleisha Kropf. Photo by Carolyn Cole / Los Angeles Times via Getty Images. Printed with permission.

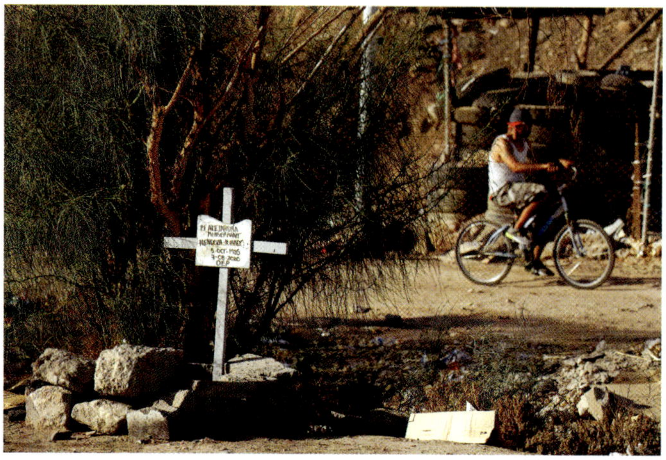

APHA
AMERICAN PUBLIC HEALTH ASSOCIATION
For science. For action. For health.

Promoting public health research, policy, practice, and education is the *AJPH* mission. As we widen our scope to embrace global issues, we also sharpen our focus to support the needs of public health practitioners. We invite contributions of original unpublished research, opinion and commentary, and letters to the editor.

The *Journal* is printed on acid-free recycled paper.

AJPH July 2024, Vol. 114, No. 7

OPEN ACCESS ONLINE ONLY PODCAST DATA SUPPLEMENT AVAILABLE

EDITOR'S CHOICE

661 Public Health Surveillance, Monitoring, or Data? Time to Decide
A. Morabia, N. Dasgupta, and L. Thorpe

BOOKS & MEDIA

663 Masterful History Tour: How and Why the Public Health Approach to Disease Has Evolved and Improved
H. Blackburn

OPINIONS, IDEAS, & PRACTICE

EDITORIALS

666 Racial/Ethnic Disparities in Pregnancy-Associated Death: The Critical Importance of Disaggregation by Cause of Death and Race/Ethnicity
C. C. Brown and D. DuBois

669 Minority Stress and Intersectionality in LGBTQIA+ Youth Mental Health Disparities
G. L. Ream

672 Safeguarding the Health of Mothers: A Public Health of Consequence, July 2024
F. Kapadia

PERSPECTIVES

674 100 Years of APHA's Public Health Education and Health Promotion Section: Honoring the Legacy of Evart G. Routzahn
M. Alperin, M. E. Auld, A. Mickalide, R. A. Galer-Unti, and M. M. Jones

679 Addressing Misinformation: A More Nuanced Understanding for Public Health Professionals
R. Wykoff, D. Harker, and L. Loveday

682 The Untapped Potential of Precision Health to Improve Heat Resilience for Those Who Need It Most
A. S. Bernstein, J. R. Malits, and G. A. Wellenius

NOTES FROM THE FIELD

685 Listening Sessions to Shape the Innovative NIH ComPASS Common Fund Program to Advance Health Equity
A. G. M. Brown, D. Winchester, S. A. Bynum, S. M. Amolegbe, Y. O. Ferguson, M. Flournoy Floyd, C. Lawhorn, J. T. Le, J. Lloyd, A. Y. Oh, N. Tyus, D. E. Whitaker, and C. A. Boyce

OPIOIDS, COVID-19, & FATAL OVERDOSES

690 Restoring and Expanding Pandemic-Era Support Policies to Reduce Economic Precarity and Overdose Deaths
A. Macmadu

693 Expanding Access to Medications for Opioid Use Disorder: Federal Policy Is Only a Part of the Solution
O. Heidari and C. J. Banta-Green

RESEARCH & ANALYSIS

OPIOIDS, COVID-19, & FATAL OVERDOSES

696 Federal Impacts on Buprenorphine Prescribing in Washington State, 2012 to 2022
F. Xiong, J. Jetson, C. Park, and C. Delcher

705 Spatial Heterogeneity in Fatal Overdose Rate Trends in Mexican Cities: 2005–2021
R. M. Henson, P. H. Mullachery, A. Sánchez-Pájaro, C. Cruz-Cruz, U. Bilal, B. Langellier, and T. Barrientos-Gutiérrez

714 State COVID-19 Policies and Drug Overdose Mortality Among Working-Age Adults in the United States, 2020
D. A. Wolf, S. M. Monnat, E. E. Wiemers, Y. Sun, X. Zhang, E. R. Grossman, and J. K. Montez

HISTORY

723 Convivial Populations: Ivan Illich and Public Health in the 21st Century
A. H. Petriceks

HEALTH MONITORING

729 Black Americans' Drug Mortality Increases and Local Employment Opportunities, 2010–2021
S. Oh and M. Cano

OPEN-THEMED RESEARCH

733 Changes in Racial and Ethnic Inequities in Pregnancy-Associated Death in the United States During the COVID-19 Pandemic
C. E. Margerison, X. Wang, S. Goldman-Mellor, M. Muzik, and A. Gemmill

BACKMATTER

ERRATA

743 Erratum In: "Characterizing the Burden of Occupational Chemical Exposures by Sociodemographic Groups in the United States, 2021"

746 Erratum In: "Airborne Lead Exposure and Childhood Cognition: The Environmental Influences on Child Health Outcomes (ECHO) Cohort (2003–2022)"

OTHER DEPARTMENTS

752 Subscription Form

Public Health Surveillance, Monitoring, or Data? Time to Decide

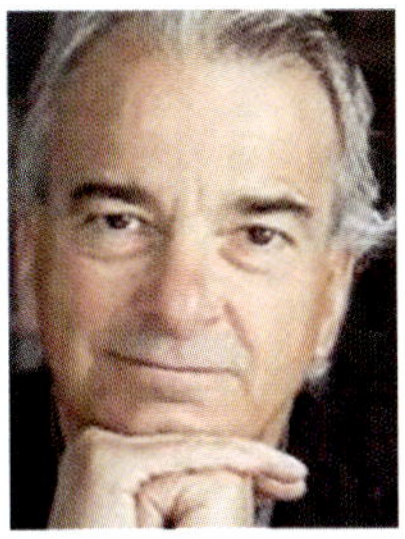
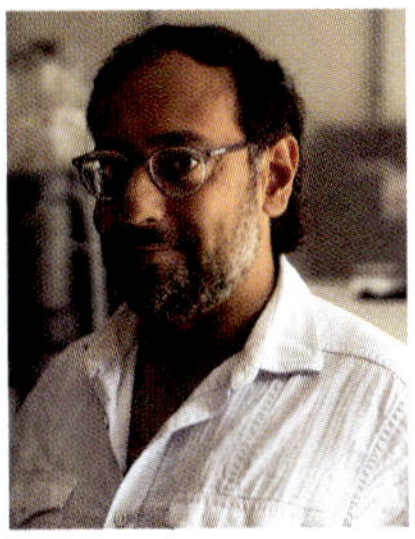
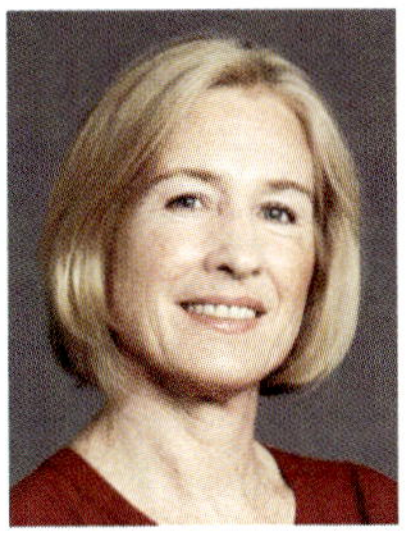

Alfredo Morabia, MD, PhD
Editor-in-Chief, *AJPH*
Nabarun Dasgupta, PhD, MPH
Associate Editor, *AJPH*
Lorna Thorpe, PhD
Associate Editor, *AJPH*

The vital role of systematically gathering population data to monitor population health is a widely held public health tenet (https://bit.ly/4bmonQu). Without these essential tools, public health professionals are often rudderless (https://bit.ly/4a8H891). With that context in mind, we bring to your attention a semantic issue of importance to our field and ask for your input.

In the October 2023 issue of the Journal, Kassler and Bowman eloquently outlined why the term "surveillance" has proven to be an unfortunate choice within the realm of public health (https://bit.ly/3Uvcot5).[3] Among the many reasons cited is the fact that "surveillance" is jargonistic and often misconstrued as a form of police activity or spying. Presently, the work is also linked to big tech tracking of consumer information for marketing purposes. Surveillance systems are also rooted in the needs of military emergency management, which prioritize immediate action over a deeper understanding of drivers of population heath (https://bit.ly/4dnqWDT; https://ojs.library.queensu.ca/index.php/surveillance-and-society/article/view/3251). "Syndromic surveillance" systems have been criticized because the practice "prioritizes standardized and transportable knowledge over local and context-dependent knowledge" (https://www.mdpi.com/2075-4698/4/3/399).

More than ever, it is our pressing duty to eliminate barriers that hinder trust between the public and public health authorities. The use of jargon and vague terminology serves to create unnecessary divisions when public health efforts should be inclusive and accessible to all.

For several months, *AJPH* has advocated adopting the term "public health monitoring" in lieu of "public health surveillance" (https://bit.ly/3UYIWxj; https://bit.ly/3y8QhkM). Public health monitoring encompasses the systematic collection of population data aimed at tracking the health status of

Continued on page e2...

HISTORY CORNER

15 YEARS AGO

Naloxone, an opioid antagonist, reverses opioid overdose by displacing opioid agonists, such as heroin or oxycodone, from opioid receptors. It is the standard treatment used by medical personnel. It has no abuse potential, and its only contraindication is a prior allergic reaction, which is rare. Although typically administered intravenously or intramuscularly, it can be administered intranasally. Strong interest in overdose prevention training and access to naloxone exists among potential overdose bystanders, including family members and drug-using partners. Overdose prevention programs with naloxone distribution that train and distribute naloxone to people who are likely to witness an overdose have been successfully implemented in several communities, including Chicago, New York, San Francisco, Baltimore, and New Mexico. . . . [The Boston Public Health Commission] naloxone distribution program is a feasible, successful program that includes distribution of intranasal naloxone by nonmedical staff. The Massachusetts Department of Public Health has identified overdose prevention as a major focus area for new public health initiatives and has expanded the program to 5 additional sites that target needle-exchange participants, staff at substance abuse treatment programs, homeless shelters, and families and friends of opioid users.

From *AJPH*, May 2009, pp. 788, 790

populations. We have now officially updated our Instructions for Authors to encourage the systematic and consistent use of this terminology (https://bit.ly/3UWezHI).

We note that the term "monitoring" is not entirely free of negative connotations either, even if these are not as readily apparent. In the context of global public health, "monitoring" may evoke systems of oversight established during colonialism: activities of grantees in low-resource settings are "monitored" by donors in wealthier countries who have little knowledge of local context (https://bit.ly/3y0mElt). Monitoring also has the taint of law enforcement punishment, specifically the practice of location-tracking devices affixed like shackles onto the ankles of parolees. The commonality across these diverse settings is that information is extracted for the benefit of authority powers at the expense of local expertise (https://bit.ly/3UsxBUB).

But "monitoring" is still less likely than "surveillance" to evoke encroachment of confidentiality. And broadly, "monitoring" is already widely used in reference to ongoing process metrics during intervention implementation.

In public health, there are powerful and valid reasons for collecting population-level data. Paying careful attention to the language used for these activities is important. Yet, changing language alone will not fix the fundamental imbalance of power that comes from existing systems of health data collection. Addressing and balancing issues of confidentiality, equitable access to data, and communicating purpose are equally important. We acknowledge that merely changing a term does not address these concerns.

Current public health monitoring systems in the United States are in dire need of a significant overhaul, a matter that former Centers for Disease Control and Prevention Director Rochelle Walensky intended to address (https://bit.ly/4dlHwns). Such a system must prioritize "privacy by design and by default," employing privacy-enhancing technologies to safeguard confidentiality and trust. At the same time, more participatory models must be developed whereby power and interpretation are returned to the people who are subjected to monitoring.

As "public health surveillance" remains the most commonly used term among public health professionals, we open a conversation with our readers, and invite comment on the use of "public health monitoring" instead of "public health surveillance" or even "public health data." Editorials of 1500 words or less (15 free references) need to be submitted by September 1, 2024, and will be considered for publication in the January 2025 issue of *AJPH*. AJPH

DOI: https://doi.org/10.2105/AJPH.2024.307709

HISTORY CORNER

50 YEARS AGO

Recent Spread of Heroin Use in the United States

Is new heroin use spreading in the United States or is it declining from a single nationwide peak which occurred around 1968? The answer may be yes to both parts of the question, depending on how incidence data are viewed. Further analysis shows that the sequence of local peak use is related to city size—large cities have generally preceded small ones. There is a definite limiting relationship, so that after a given time all cities of a certain size will have experienced peak use. This relationship implies that new heroin use may continue to appear in smaller cities in the future. Currently (1974), rising heroin use incidence is limited to Standard Metropolitan Statistical Areas (SMSAs) of about 500,000 population or less. The shift from large to small is empirically similar to "hierarchical diffusion" observed in the spread of innovations (such as television). . . . These estimated results suggest the need for continuous reallocation of drug treatment funds to smaller and smaller cities as peak use shifts and treatment demands declines in areas of older heroin use.

From *AJPH*, Supplement 1, December 1974, p. 16

Masterful History Tour: How and Why the Public Health Approach to Disease Has Evolved and Improved

Henry Blackburn, MD

ABOUT THE AUTHOR

Henry Blackburn is Mayo professor emeritus, Division of Epidemiology and Community Health, School of Public Health, University of Minnesota, Minneapolis.

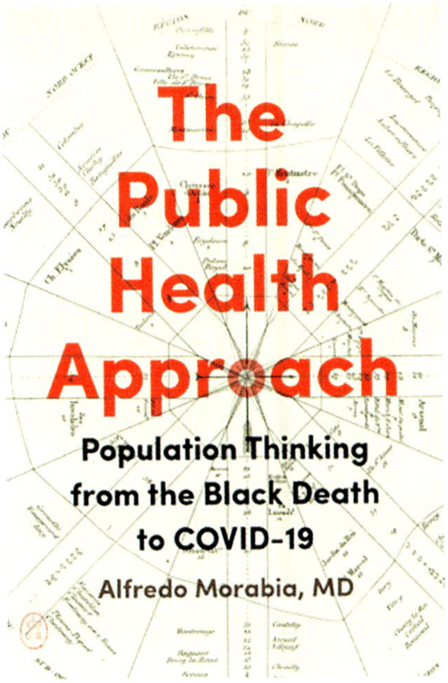

The Public Health Approach: Population Thinking From the Black Death to COVID-19
By Alfredo Morabia
Baltimore, MD: Johns Hopkins University Press; 2023
232 pp.; $29.95
ISBN-10: 1421446782
ISBN-13: 978-1421446783

Alfredo Morabia's engaging new book confronts a major controversy within medicine and fills the need for a clearer understanding of health and disease in whole populations as well as in individuals. As a physician, epidemiologist, and historian at the center of modern public health, Morabia is well-equipped to cover the evolution of a population view and public health approach from antiquity to the policy and action needed today. This fresh perspective is particularly welcome today when personalized "precision medicine" for individuals is the dominant theme in medical teaching, research, and practice. That he writes short chapters—fascinating stories about successive pandemics of civilization and with rich insights—represents mastery of thinking, organization, and writing.

WHAT IS "POPULATION THINKING"?

Morabia notes that people usually cite individual experiences in arriving at their understanding of health and disease. But anecdotal information about one or a few cases is not helpful in assessing health status or making recommendations for an entire society. A population view, on the other hand, allows useful comparisons and even predictions when systematic measurements of physical and behavioral characteristics among representative groups across varied cultures are followed for subsequent rates of disease and death.[1(p3)]

THE PANDEMIC CHAPTERS

Although an appendix to the book delves into "Precursors to Population Thinking" gleaned from ancient literature, Morabia posits that the first great departure from medicine's preoccupation with sick individuals came with the plague—the Black Death of the 16th century. England's Henry VIII quarantined its ports but also ordered local officials to report each week "how many had died and whereof they died."[1(p23)] The Weekly Bills of Mortality—quantitative data collected in a similar fashion over time—"provided the platform for a shift to population thinking . . . a decisive first step in public health science."[1(p24)]

By the 17th century, John Graunt, a haberdasher and perhaps the first demographer and epidemiologist, recognized "astonishing regularities" in London deaths per year, which allowed prompt recognition of and potential explanations for irregularities. Morabia considers Graunt's analyses of the reports in his 1662 *National and Political Observations on the Bills of Mortality*,[2] as "the common ancestor of all population-based sciences . . . statistics, epidemiology, sociology, and demography."[1(p36)]

AJPH July 2024, Vol. 114, No. 7

It was not until the 18th-century smallpox epidemic in the American colonies that a sound public health approach was established, comparing vaccinated and unvaccinated cohorts. Benjamin Franklin and Cotton Mather promoted vaccination throughout the colonies; it even became a factor in the success of American troops during the Revolutionary War. Eventually, in 1980, the World Health Organization vaccination campaign could proclaim elimination of smallpox infection.[1(p51)]

A report on the devastating Paris cholera epidemic of 1829–1833 was a methodological advance in analyzing mortality data according to age and gender. But because "sanitary reformers" identified "miasma" (foul air) as the origin of the disease, their strategies against it—including sweeping filth from streets into the river—were counterproductive. The common source was the contaminated River Seine!

A breakthrough for population thinking came with an 1850 London Epidemiological Society conference on cholera. Its "contagionist" conferees were the first to differentiate effects of polluted water from those of air pollution and successfully link population-based research to public health policy.[1(p62)]

During the 1854 London epidemic, before identification of the organism that causes cholera, physician John Snow drew his now well-known conclusions relating infections from pumps delivering water from the nearby polluted Thames compared with pumps providing water from the cleaner river upstream.[3] Competition continued, nevertheless, between forces promoting "sanitary reforms" and specialists of a new public health science, including bacteriology. By the end of the 19th century, bacteriology prevailed. The argument of miasma versus germs was over.

The 19th- and early 20th-century pandemic of pulmonary tuberculosis (TB) was a problem for diagnosis and control because of the latent period between acquiring infection and developing symptoms, a chronic clinical course, and a lack of specific therapy. "Consumption" was better controlled in 1945 after a randomized clinical trial of treatment with streptomycin showed dramatic effects on TB mortality, a trial that profoundly affected clinical medicine and public health.[4]

Advances in noncommunicable-disease epidemiology were part of enhanced population thinking following World War II with the burgeoning epidemics of cardiovascular disease (CVD) and chronic pulmonary disease and cancer. Multiple, often socially determined risk factors were identified in these and other cohort studies:

- the 1948 Framingham Heart Study—a long-term, community-wide approach defining individual CVD risk[5];
- the 1950 British Doctors Study of air pollution and tobacco smoking in relation to chronic pulmonary disease and lung cancer[6]; and
- the 1957 Seven Countries Study among mainly rural cohorts of all working men aged 40 to 59 years residing in areas thought to contrast in traditional diet or in rate of heart attack.[7,8]

Morabia credits British physician-epidemiologist Geoffrey Rose with groundbreaking population thinking when, using data from these cohort studies, he showed that only a small proportion of heart attacks arose from the fraction having "abnormal" levels of blood cholesterol. Rather, most cases came from the large central part of the population distribution of cholesterol. He also demonstrated that the frequency of "high-risk" individuals in a population is fixed to the mean of its risk factor levels; thus, lowering the mean would greatly benefit the entire population; it would offer little advantage to any individual. Rose labeled this the "prevention paradox."[9]

The advent of pandemic HIV/AIDS in the early 1980s presented new research challenges. With the low incidence in Western countries making mass screening unwieldy and inaccurate, AIDS researchers turned attention to trial design. Ultimately, the analyses of AIDS cause and treatment became part of "a new conceptual framework that resulted in refinement of the Public Health Approach."[1(p105)]

Morabia notes that while the influenza epidemic of 1918 demonstrated inadequacy of international planning and preparation for infectious disease outbreaks, COVID-19 indicated how little the world's surveillance and reporting systems had improved in the 100 years between these pandemics. He acknowledges that leaders among today's vulnerable populations were more ready to develop vaccines and promote healthy behaviors but expresses concern about the increasingly negative role of "tribal politics," "fake news," and loss of trust in science, government, and the press. "Preparing for future pandemics requires a vibrant health monitoring system," he writes. "The future of the Public Health Approach depends on it."[1(p129)]

SOCIAL DETERMINANTS OF HEALTH

In addition to the concepts of "population thinking" and the "public

AJPH July 2024, Vol. 114, No. 7

health approach," Morabia submits "social determinants" as another lens through which to view large-scale causes and consequences of disease. This idea emerged over the course of the post–World War II cohort studies that established the risk factors for epidemic CVD and cancers, including levels of blood pressure and blood cholesterol and the number of cigarettes smoked daily. These began to be considered in terms of the social culture that influences them: "aspects of the economy, education, health care, and the social and built environments."[1(p108)]

Postwar society saw many social changes toward urbanization, less work and leisure-time physical activity, more motor transport, more cigarette smoking, and eating patterns rich in animal products and calories. Morabia writes, "It looked like these diseases were consequences of the modern way of life."[1(p107)] In this valuable chapter (Chapter 8), he places modern health problems squarely in the context of social inequities, pointing out that risk is not the same in every social stratum and challenging the assumption that individuals are responsible for their disadvantages when the causes are societal. His listing of current social issues arising from "unequal access to essential human needs" includes occupational stress and unhealthful working conditions; civil rights violations; mistreatment by police; drug and alcohol addiction; discrimination against racial, ethnic, and sexual minorities; and racially disproportionate incarceration.

Rising mortality trends and falling life expectancy of US populations drew the attention of Woolf et al., who write, "The wide range of affected conditions points to the need to examine *systemic* causes of declining health in the U.S. [italics added]"[1(p117)]

EPILOGUE: THE PUBLIC HEALTH APPROACH

Having demonstrated that individual health outcomes are closely tied to the health of the population, Morabia sums up:

> Doctors give prescriptions to individuals who are free to comply with them or not, but a public health recommendation is a collective response to a collective threat. For the public health approach to be effective, everyone in the population must know about it and have access to its benefits. . . . Individually, we are powerless against these scourges.[1(p144–145)]

This volume will be enjoyed by and will enrich the understanding of a wide readership, including students, scholars, and historians of science, medicine, public health, the humanities, and communications, as well as the intelligent general reader. AJPH

CORRESPONDENCE

Correspondence should be sent to Henry Blackburn, MD, Division of Epidemiology and Community Health, School of Public Health, University of Minnesota, 1300 Second St S Suite 300, Minneapolis, MN 55454 (e-mail: black002@umn.edu). Reprints can be ordered at https://ajph.org by clicking the "Reprints" link.

PUBLICATION INFORMATION

Full Citation: Blackburn H. Masterful history tour: how and why the public health approach to disease has evolved and improved. *Am J Public Health*. 2024;114(7):663–665.

Acceptance Date: January 31, 2024.

DOI: https://doi.org/10.2105/AJPH.2024.307600

CONFLICTS OF INTEREST

The author reports no conflicts of interest.

REFERENCES

1. Morabia A. *The Public Health Approach: Population Thinking From the Black Death to COVID-19*. Baltimore, MD: Johns Hopkins University Press; 2023. https://doi.org/10.56021/9781421446783
2. Graunt, J. *Natural and Political Observations Made Upon the Bills of Mortality, 1662*. Wilcox WJ, ed. Baltimore, MD: Johns Hopkins University Press; 1939.
3. Snow J. *Snow on Cholera*. New York, NY: The Commonwealth Fund; 1936:97–98.
4. Streptomycin treatment of pulmonary tuberculosis: a Medical Research Council Investigation. *BMJ*. 1948;2(4582):769–782. https://doi.org/10.1136/bmj.2.4582.769
5. Dawber TR, Moore FE, Mann GV. Coronary heart disease in the Framingham Heart Study. *Am J Public Health*. 1957;47(4/2):4–24. https://doi.org/10.2105/AJPH.47.4_Pt_2.4.
6. Doll R, Hill AB. The mortality of doctors in relation to their smoking habits. A preliminary report. *BMJ*. 1954;1(4877):1451–1455. https://doi.org/10.1136/bmj.1.4877.1451
7. Keys A, Blackburn H, Menotti A, et al. Coronary heart disease in seven countries. *Circulation*. 1970;41(suppl 1):1–211.
8. University of Minnesota. Heart attack prevention. A history of cardiovascular disease epidemiology, 1945 to 1975. Available at: http://www.epi.umn.edu/cvdepi. Accessed January 12, 2024.
9. Rose G. *The Strategy of Preventive Medicine*. New York, NY: Oxford University Press; 1993. https://doi.org/10.1093/oso/9780192624864.001.0001

Racial/Ethnic Disparities in Pregnancy-Associated Death: The Critical Importance of Disaggregation by Cause of Death and Race/Ethnicity

Clare C. Brown, PhD, MPH, and Dominique DuBois, RN

ABOUT THE AUTHORS

Clare C. Brown is with the Fay W. Boozman College of Public Health, University of Arkansas for Medical Sciences, Little Rock. Dominique DuBois is with the College of Nursing, University of Arkansas for Medical Sciences.

See also Margerison et al., p. 733.

AJPH July 2024, Vol. 114, No. 7

Racial/ethnic disparities in perinatal health outcomes are among the most widely recognized, long-standing health inequities in the United States, with more than double the rate of pregnancy-related mortality among non-Hispanic Native Hawaiian or Other Pacific Islander (NHOPI; 62.8 deaths per 100 000 live births), non-Hispanic Black (39.9), and non-Hispanic American Indian or Alaska Native (AIAN; 32.0) individuals than among non-Hispanic White individuals (14.1).[1] Given that 84% of pregnancy-related deaths are preventable,[2] efforts to better understand and prevent maternal death are critical for improving health equity.

Studies have reported large increases in the rates of pregnancy-related death over the past several decades; however, a pivotal evaluation from the National Center of Health Statistics, which maintains a centralized database of all death certificates in the United States, indicated that much of the recent increase in maternal mortality was largely the result of improvements in data collection because of the addition of the pregnancy checkbox on the revised standard certificate of death in 2003.[3,4] Despite the likelihood that the staggered introduction of the checkbox artificially amplified documented increases in maternal mortality, all states adopted the checkbox by 2017. The most recent analyses from the Centers for Disease Control and Prevention indicated an annual increase in the maternal mortality rate from 2018 to 2021 overall and for all three races/ethnicities studied, with larger increases for non-Hispanic Black and Hispanic individuals than for non-Hispanic White individuals.[5]

Although many evaluations do not include incidental and accidental causes in the definition of pregnancy-related death, there is a growing recognition of the contribution of incidental causes to the growth in pregnancy-associated death overall as well as the large racial/ethnic inequities in pregnancy-associated death. In this issue of *AJPH*, Margerison et al. (p. 733) evaluate changes in five categories of pregnancy-associated death during the first two years of the COVID-19 pandemic and find that nearly one of every three pregnancy-associated deaths during the study period (2018–2021) was drug, suicide, or homicide related.

However, their study highlights a much broader public health issue that goes beyond the pandemic. Specifically, the authors highlight large racial/ethnic disparities in each of the three incidental or accidental causes, irrespective of the pandemic. First, non-Hispanic AIAN individuals had four times the rate of drug-related pregnancy-associated deaths than did non-Hispanic White individuals (2021). Second, non-Hispanic Black individuals had nine times the rate of pregnancy-associated deaths from homicide than did non-Hispanic White individuals (2020–2021). Third, NHOPI individuals had nearly six times the rate of pregnancy-associated deaths from suicide than non-Hispanic White individuals (2020–2021).

It is critical that policymakers and public health officials continue to address the high rates of pregnancy-associated death related to suicide, homicide, and drug overdose. Estimates of preventability of maternal mortality vary depending on the report; however, a recent study of data from 14 state maternal mortality review committees found that although 68% of maternal deaths were preventable, intervention could have prevented 100% of maternal deaths attributable to mental health conditions, including substance use disorders.[6] Continued efforts to ensure culturally congruent screening and treatment across a broad range of mental health conditions and substance use disorders are critically needed throughout the pregnancy and postpartum periods.

Margerison et al. describe the significant increases in different types of pregnancy-associated deaths during the first two years of the pandemic, highlighting that the increased inequities in obstetric-, drug-, and homicide-related causes of pregnancy-associated deaths were likely a result of the exacerbation of many existing structural and systematic inequities during the COVID-19 pandemic. Despite the importance of the findings specific to COVID-19 and the implications for addressing the long-standing racial/ethnic inequities in maternal mortality, Margerison et al. provide a template for evaluations of inequities outside the perinatal space.

Maternal mortality is a relatively rare outcome, with a small number of occurrences of maternal death for some racial/ethnic groups in a given year, particularly when stratifying by the type or cause of maternal death. Margerison et al. made a conscious, well-explained effort to provide findings for each of the defined types of maternal death for all available racial/ethnic categories available in the data, regardless of the number of deaths. The authors additionally take the time to carefully explain the purpose of including rates of pregnancy-associated death for all racial/ethnic groups and make clear notations in the figures and tables of small numerator (i.e., death) counts. For the particularly rare types of pregnancy-associated death (i.e., homicide, suicide, and other causes), the authors opted to aggregate two years of data rather than aggregating multiple races/ethnicities or mortality types.

Researchers are often inclined to remove small subgroups from subgroup analyses or to aggregate subgroups together (e.g., an "other race" category) to ensure adequate sample size. Such approaches largely stem from the need to ensure adequate sample size to meet normal distribution assumptions of many statistical tests, as well as to protect the privacy of the individuals. In their study, Margerison et al. highlight that small numerator death counts may limit some statistical testing, yet exclusion of findings for a given race or ethnicity because of a small number of deaths may mask critical health inequities. This ultimately weakens the ability to focus on associated populations and allocate resources accordingly. Such "data genocide" is not an entirely novel concept, as it was brought to the forefront during the COVID-19 pandemic when failure to collect timely, detailed racial/ethnic data in many states often led to unavailable surveillance metrics for AIAN populations.[7–9]

In the study by Margerison et al., some of the primary study findings would have been completely absent if the study excluded findings for racial/ethnic subgroups with relatively few pregnancy-associated deaths of certain causes. For example, whereas obstetric pregnancy-associated death increased by approximately 28% from 2019 to 2020 overall, the rate more than doubled for NHOPI individuals (from 39.3 to 94.2 per 100 000 live births). Additionally, providing rates of drug-related pregnancy deaths among AIAN individuals for each year highlighted the stark increases in drug-related pregnancy-associated deaths among AIAN individuals in 2021.

Consequently, although the study by Margerison et al. has important implications for maternal health, their evaluation has much broader importance for the field of health equity. We as researchers, journal reviewers, teachers, and public health and clinical practitioners must make efforts to recognize the importance of disaggregating findings for all races/ethnicities when such information is available. Disaggregation of findings by race/ethnicity is important for ensuring that data are readily available for all populations, particularly historically marginalized populations who face high rates of adverse outcomes despite the relatively small number of individuals in the numerator. Although it is important to ensure that the use of such disaggregated subpopulations does not allow re-identification or facilitate racial or ethnic targeting,[10] failure to provide outcomes for all available races/ethnicities, when analytically appropriate, may result in the inability to detect and address important health inequities. As shown in this study, careful consideration of all racial/ethnic subgroups can provide valuable insight for policymaking and resource allocation efforts aimed at improving health equity. AJPH

CORRESPONDENCE

Correspondence should be sent to Clare C. Brown, University of Arkansas for Medical Sciences, 4301 W Markham St, Slot #812, Little Rock, AR 72205-7199 (e-mail: cbrown3@uams.edu). Reprints can be ordered at http://www.ajph.org by clicking the "Reprints" link.

PUBLICATION INFORMATION

Full Citation: Brown CC, DuBois D. Racial/ethnic disparities in pregnancy-associated death: the critical importance of disaggregation by cause of death and race/ethnicity. *Am J Public Health*. 2024;114(7):666–668.

Acceptance Date: April 15, 2024.

DOI: https://doi.org/10.2105/AJPH.2024.307700

ORCID iD:
Clare C. Brown https://orcid.org/0000-0001-7149-4739

CONTRIBUTORS

Both authors wrote and revised the editorial.

ACKNOWLEDGMENTS

C. C. Brown was supported by the National Institute on Minority Health and Health Disparities (NIMHD) of the National Institutes of Health (grant 1K01MD018072). D. DuBois received funding from the Arkansas Center for Health Disparities T32 Predoctoral Training Program (grant T32 MD015016), which is supported by the NIMHD.

Note. The content of this editorial is solely the responsibility of the authors and does not necessarily represent the official views of the funders. Funders had no role in the design, analysis, or writing of this article.

CONFLICTS OF INTEREST

The authors have no conflicts of interest to report.

REFERENCES

1. Centers for Disease Control and Prevention. Pregnancy mortality surveillance system. 2023. Available at: https://www.cdc.gov/reproductivehealth/maternal-mortality/pregnancy-mortality-surveillance-system.htm. Accessed March 11, 2024.
2. Trost S, Beauregard J, Chandra G, et al. Pregnancy-related deaths: data from maternal mortality review committees in 36 US states, 2017–2019. 2022. Available at: https://www.cdc.gov/reproductivehealth/maternal-mortality/docs/pdf/Pregnancy-Related-Deaths-Data-MMRCs-2017-2019-H.pdf. Accessed April 22, 2024.
3. Rossen LM, Womack LS, Hoyert DL, Anderson RN, Uddin SFG. The impact of the pregnancy checkbox and misclassification on maternal mortality trends in the United States, 1999–2017. *Vital Health Stat 3*. 2020;(44):1–61.
4. Joseph KS, Boutin A, Lisonkova S, et al. Maternal mortality in the United States: recent trends, current status, and future considerations. *Obstet Gynecol*. 2021;137(5):763–771. https://doi.org/10.1097/AOG.0000000000004361
5. Hoyert DL. Maternal mortality rates in the United States, 2021. March 16, 2023. https://doi.org/10.15620/cdc:124678
6. Trost SL, Beauregard JL, Smoots AN, et al. Preventing pregnancy-related mental health deaths: insights from 14 US maternal mortality review committees, 2008–17. *Health Aff (Millwood)*. 2021;40(10):1551–1559. https://doi.org/10.1377/hlthaff.2021.00615
7. Urban Indian Health Institute. Data genocide of American Indians and Alaska Natives in COVID-19 data. February 15, 2021. Available at: https://www.uihi.org/projects/data-genocide-of-american-indians-and-alaska-natives-in-covid-19-data. Accessed April 22, 2024.
8. Huyser KR, Horse AJY, Kuhlemeier AA, Huyser MR. COVID-19 pandemic and Indigenous representation in public health data. *Am J Public Health*. 2021;111(suppl 3):S208–S214. https://doi.org/10.2105/AJPH.2021.306415
9. Nguyen KH, Lew KP, Trivedi AN. Trends in collection of disaggregated Asian American, Native Hawaiian, and Pacific Islander data: opportunities in federal health surveys. *Am J Public Health*. 2022;112(10):1429–1435. https://doi.org/10.2105/AJPH.2022.306969
10. Kader F, Doan LN, Lee M, Chin MK, Kwon SC, Yi SS. Disaggregating race/ethnicity data categories: criticisms, dangers, and opposing viewpoints. *Health Affairs Forefront*. March 25, 2022. https://doi.org/10.1377/forefront.20220323.555023.

Minority Stress and Intersectionality in LGBTQIA+ Youth Mental Health Disparities

Geoffrey L. Ream, PhD

ABOUT THE AUTHOR

Geoffrey L. Ream is a professor at the Adelphi University School of Social Work, Garden City, NY.

Note. *The opinions expressed in this work are those of the author and do not necessarily represent those of Adelphi University or any other organization.*

The article by Beccia et al.[1] is one of several recent works that utilize intersectionality together with minority stress theory to analyze lesbian, gay, bisexual, transgender, queer, questioning, intersex, asexual, aromantic, nonbinary, and other minoritized sexual and gender identity (LGBTQIA+) versus non-LGBTQIA+ mental health disparities. Intersectionality, as described by Beccia et al.,[1] originated with Black feminism, and it describes how interacting dynamics of power and privilege shape experiences at various intersections of race, gender, sexual orientation, urbanicity, and other demographic characteristics. Minority stress became a prevailing theory in LGBTQIA+ psychology in the early 2000s, during the "Culture Wars." Minority stress holds that LGBTQIA+ health disparities exist because of the manifold effects of stigma and discrimination at all levels of society. Minority stress counters a narrative still promulgated by anti-LGBTQIA+ political and religious forces that LGBTQIA+ health disparities exist because of some inherent pathology associated with being LGBTQIA+.[2] Beccia et al.[1] discussed LGBTQIA+ adult mental health, and this editorial describes how minority stress and intersectionality apply to LGBTQIA+ youth mental health, with some suggestions for future directions.

Applying intersectionality to LGBTQIA+ mental health has become much more feasible recently since panel studies and government databases started including the necessary variables, as alluded to by Beccia et al.[1] The Centers for Disease Control and Prevention started coding for sexual orientation and transgender identity in its National Violent Death Reporting System (NVDRS)[2] during the 2010s, at the request of research, practice, and advocacy organizations. The Youth Risk Behavior Survey (YRBS),[3] featured in several recent studies on LGBTQIA+ mental health, started including sexual orientation questions in its national survey in 2015.

RACE AND LGBTQIA+ IDENTITY

Once they have the data, researchers can explore unique effects at the intersections of race, sexual orientation, and gender. These have turned out to be many and varied. Some recent findings suggest that LGBTQIA+ youths of color may be partially inoculated against mental health risk from anti-LGBTQIA+ oppression because they are taught resiliency against racial oppression from an early age.[3] Alternatively, LGBTQIA+ youth of color may be at higher risk because parents and others involved with children in their communities strictly police nonnormative sexuality and gender expression on grounds that oppressors might use it as evidence to support their stereotype that the whole community is sexually deviant.[4] Groups that have LGBTQIA+-tolerant narratives woven into their history may be affected by generations of oppression and normalized maladaptive coping, leading to lower resiliency for LGBTQIA+ youths and everyone else.[5] Entire national governments, guided by traditional values that are not necessarily religious, may disallow formation of organizations that would push for LGBTQIA+ supportive environments in schools, with predictable effects on LGBTQIA+ youths' mental health.[6] Especially high levels of lifetime risk can be found among LGBTQIA+ graduates of home schools, the signature initiative of the well-resourced and globally powerful evangelical Christian movement, which "protects" youth from LGBTQIA+-affirming influences that could reach them via schools or the Internet.[1,7]

As Beccia et al. suggest, the combination of minority stress and intersectionality can also help in designing and assessing interventions. A program based on trending personal narrative videos about difficulty in adolescence and freedom in young adulthood may have mixed results, and might even be unhelpful, among adolescents who see few faces or body types like theirs in the videos and will not gain much additional control over their circumstances in the transition to young adulthood.[8] A powerful source of resilience, albeit mostly for its target demographic, may be found in a "kiki" scene organized by and for urban Black LGBTQIA+ youths, who use the space to develop their social networks and self-expressions outside of the competitive environment of the house balls.[9]

Minority stress and intersectionality can also help describe LGBTQIA+ youths' complex relationships with social institutions that both help and harm in turn. Hegemonic conservative religion can be problematic on the macro level because it promulgates anti-LGBTQIA+ ideologies in a space where they are hard to debunk with modern science. Religion can be relatively helpful on the micro level, however, because it discourages overt individual-level anti-LGBTQIA+ abusiveness.[10]

One key opportunity for research on LGBTQIA+ youth mental health disparities lies in that sources like YRBS and NVDRS now have enough data including sexual orientation variables to assess trends over time. In his preface to the paperback edition of *Stamped From the Beginning* (2016), Ibram X. Kendi described racism and antiracism as "dual and dueling" social forces throughout American history, with progress on one side often followed by progress on the other.[11(p.x)] The same can be said of anti-LGBTQIA+ and LGBTQIA+-affirming movements, whose efforts in the policy, practice, and cultural realms have predictable negative and positive effects on LGBTQIA+ youths' mental health. These effects emerge in analyses of public health data. YRBS, NVDRS, and similar data sources with indicators for broad demographic categories can suggest where problems are and where they might be growing, and more targeted investigations can connect issues to specific demographics, historical moments, and social forces.

GENERATIONAL DIFFERENCES

Data on trends over time can be used to assess generational effects. Generation Z are the characteristically online "Zoomers," who grew up with unprecedented access to LGBTQIA+-affirming discourse spaces. Earlier generations of survey researchers wondered whether the "one in 10" political talking point might reflect an overestimate, but current polls show that 28% of Generation Z identifies as LGBTQIA+.[12] COVID-19 forcing everyone online coincided with significant advances in discourse on LGBTQIA+ issues, specifically around asexuality, aromanticism, agender, and nonbinary gender. Many people who identified as lesbian, gay, bisexual, or transgender report a second, more authentic coming out experience after finding this discourse, with predictable improvements to their mental health. However, long hours of social media use come with known risks of problem use patterns and exposure to cyberbullying. Better technology and fewer boundaries around accessing it in the home can intensify these risks. Generation Z voices on YouTube describe a trajectory of parasocial relationships replacing social relationships, and then both being replaced by simply passively consuming media, often in a fantasy frame of reference. Time spent this way is time not spent pursuing career, romantic, identity, or health goals.

Generation Z also struggles with mental health. They are the "lockdown generation" who lived with school lockdown drills under the threat of mass shooters for years before being actually locked down because of COVID-19. They are now presenting on college campuses, and presumably at workplaces, with higher rates of mental health risk factors than research used to attribute just to LGBTQIA+ youths. In a June 2022 survey, 60% of college students reported having been diagnosed with a mental illness by a professional.[13] Mental health disparities research on post–COVID-19 LGBTQIA+ youths should recognize that it compares them to a baseline in which the kids are not all right.

FUTURE DIRECTIONS

Effects of pandemic stress, race, gender, LGBTQIA+ identity, historical oppression, recent anti-LGBTQIA+ policies, generation-wide issues, online-ness, specific sources of resiliency, and experiences with interventions will likely all emerge in the data on LGBTQIA+ youth mental health disparities after COVID-19 that are now becoming available. It will be hard for any one study to parse them all. Minority stress and intersectionality can help organize this work so that the findings taken together will form an updated, nuanced picture of post–COVID-19 LGBTQIA+ youths' mental health. AJPH

CORRESPONDENCE

Correspondence should be sent to Geoffrey L. Ream, Adelphi University, School of Social Work, PO Box 701, Garden City, NY 11530 (e-mail: ream@adelphi.edu). Reprints can be ordered at https://ajph.org by clicking the "Reprints" link.

PUBLICATION INFORMATION

Full Citation: Ream GL. Minority stress and intersectionality in LGBTQIA+ youth mental health disparities. *Am J Public Health*. 2024;114(7):669–671.

Acceptance Date: March 25, 2024.

DOI: https://doi.org/10.2105/AJPH.2024.307676

CONFLICTS OF INTEREST

The author reports no conflicts of interest.

REFERENCES

1. Beccia A, Zubizarreta D, Austin SB, Raifman JR, Chavarro JE, Charlton BM. Trajectories of mental distress among US women by sexual orientation and racialized group during the first year of the COVID-19 pandemic. *Am J Public Health*.

2024;114(5):511–522. https://doi.org/10.2105/AJPH.2024.307601

2. Ream GL. Trends in deaths by suicide 2014–2019 among lesbian, gay, bisexual, transgender, queer, questioning, and other gender/sexual minority (LGBTQ+) youth. *J Adolesc Health.* 2022;71(5):609–615. https://doi.org/10.1016/j.jadohealth.2022.06.017
3. Rosales R, Sellers CM, Lee CS, Santos B, O'Brien K, Colby SM. Examining racial/ethnic differences in the association of victimization and suicidal thoughts and behaviors with alcohol use among sexual minority youth. *LGBT Health.* 2023;10(2):109–120. https://doi.org/10.1089/lgbt.2021.0267
4. Stanford A. *Homophobia in the Black Church: How Faith, Politics, and Fear Divide the Black Community.* Santa Barbara, CA: Praeger; 2013. https://doi.org/10.5040/9798400666278
5. Schuler A, Wedel A, Kelsey SW, et al. Suicidality by sexual identity and correlates among American Indian and Alaska native high school students. *J Adolesc Health.* 2023;73(6):1030–1037. https://doi.org/10.1016/j.jadohealth.2023.07.020
6. Wei C, Liu W. Coming out in Mainland China: a national survey of LGBTQ students. *J LGBT Youth.* 2019;16(2):192–219. https://doi.org/10.1080/19361653.2019.1565795
7. Anderson SO, Lough BJ. Sexual and gender minoritized youth in Christian home schools: perceptions of climate and support. *J LGBT Youth.* 2021;18(4):438–458. https://doi.org/10.1080/19361653.2019.1700404
8. Brandon-Friedman RA, Kinney MK. Does it get better? Exploring "it gets better" videos using visual sociology. *J LGBT Youth.* 2021;18(4):421–437. https://doi.org/10.1080/19361653.2019.1691107
9. Harper GW, LaBoy R, Castillo M, Johnson GL, Hosek SG, Jadwin-Cakmak L. It's a kiki!: developmental benefits of the kiki scene for Black gay/bisexual/transgender adolescents/emerging adults. *J LGBT Youth.* 2022;19(1):31–52. https://doi.org/10.1080/19361653.2020.1813672
10. Bailey BM, Heath MA, Jackson AP, et al. An ethnographic exploration of adolescent homophobic language in a rural religiously-conservative high school. *J LGBT Youth.* 2022;19(2):217–245. https://doi.org/10.1080/19361653.2020.1788479
11. Ibram X. Kendi. *Stamped from the Beginning: The Definitive History of Racist Ideas in America.* New York, NY: Nation Books; 2017
12. PRRI. A political and cultural glimpse into America's future: Generation Z's views on generational change and the challenges and opportunities ahead. 2024. Available at: https://www.prri.org/wp-content/uploads/2024/01/PRRI-Jan-2024-Gen-Z-Draft.pdf. Accessed March 28, 2024.
13. Leonhardt M. Crisis on campus: 60% of college kids are living with mental health disorders, and schools are woefully unprepared. *Fortune.* July 12, 2022. Available at: https://fortune.com/well/2022/07/12/mental-health-crisis-college-schools-unprepared. Accessed March 28, 2024.

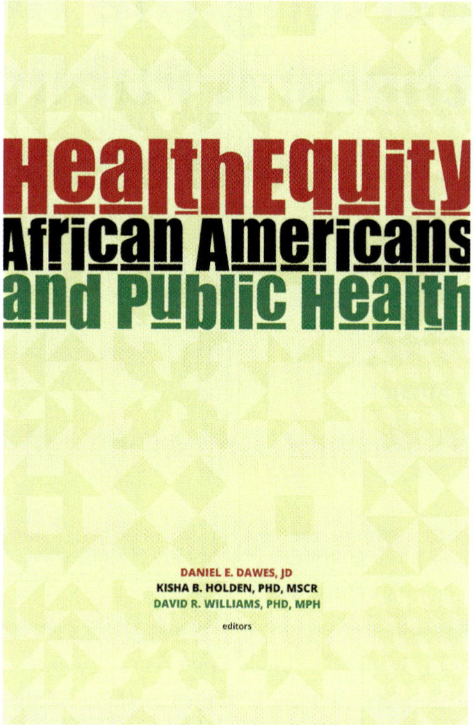

Safeguarding the Health of Mothers: A Public Health of Consequence, July 2024

Farzana Kapadia, PhD, MPH

ABOUT THE AUTHOR

Farzana Kapadia is the deputy editor of AJPH *and a professor in the Department of Epidemiology, New York University School of Global Public Health, New York.*

AJPH July 2024, Vol. 114, No. 7

Maternal mortality in the United States remains unacceptably high, irrespective of how maternal mortality estimates are calculated.[1,2] Moreover, racial/ethnic inequities in maternal mortality persist. Driven by multifactorial causes that range from individual- to structural-level factors, maternal mortality inequities are grounded in structurally racist and discriminatory access to appropriate and timely obstetric, gynecological, and primary health care.[3] More recently, inadequate Medicaid expansion across US states (https://bit.ly/4d4E68C), inconsistent extension of Medicaid coverage for postpartum care,[4] and growing antiabortion legislation[5] have further undermined efforts to reduce the inequity gaps in maternal mortality. The COVID-19 pandemic pulled back the curtain on the growing inadequacies in health care access for marginalized communities, inadequate prevention programming, and growing disparities in other causes of death from accidents and injuries.

MEASURING MATERNAL MORTALITY

The World Health Organization defines maternal deaths as "deaths from any cause related to or aggravated by pregnancy or its management (excluding accidental or incidental causes) during pregnancy and childbirth or within 42 days of termination of pregnancy, irrespective of the duration and site of the pregnancy" (https://bit.ly/3w8rLiU). To ensure accurate counting of maternal death, in 2003 the National Vital Statistics System added a checkbox to death certificates to report whether the person who died was pregnant at the time of death or had recently been pregnant. Because of the incremental, rather than uniform, uptake in use of this checkbox on death certificates across US states, some suggest that observed increases in maternal mortality are artifactual rather than real increases over time.

However, there are two issues with this interpretation of an overestimation. First, as shown in a recent Centers for Disease Control and Prevention report and as summarized by Brown and DuBois (p. 666) in this issue of *AJPH*, the rate of maternal mortality among Black people in 2021 was 69.9 deaths per 100 000 live births, which was 2.6 times the rate for White people (https://bit.ly/4aYoO3X). As these rates indicate, the United States is still not doing better than, or as well as, peer countries, and inequities in maternal mortality by race/ethnicity persist. Second—and more relevant from a public health perspective and in line with the World Health Organization definition of a maternal death—by counting all deaths of people who were pregnant at the time of death, the United States is more accurately monitoring all pregnancy-related deaths, not just deaths among those who have experienced a live birth and obtaining a more accurate reflection of the mortality risk associated with pregnancy.

PERSISTENCE OF RACIAL/ETHNIC INEQUITIES

Several Centers for Disease Control and Prevention reports identified pregnant people to be at increased risk for adverse outcomes associated with COVID-19, including pregnancy complications, severe illness, and death attributable to decreased lung capacity and a weakened immune system.[6] According to a 2022 Government Accountability Office report, COVID-19 was a contributing factor in one quarter of all maternal deaths in 2020 and 2021 (https://bit.ly/3U9tOLH). These data suggest that maternal mortality during the pandemic may have been related to COVID-19–associated complications as well as delays and disruptions to access to timely pre- and postnatal health care. Also during the pandemic, deaths resulting from overdose, violence, and other intentional and unintentional injuries increased among younger adults, including women.

Understanding the extent to which these multiple, and often reinforcing, drivers of overall mortality among people of reproductive age affected pregnancy-associated mortality (a death while pregnant or within 1 year of the end of pregnancy from any cause related to or aggravated by the pregnancy) during the COVID-19 pandemic is critical. To this end, Margerison et al. (p. 733) employed National Vital Statistics System data to examine pregnancy-associated deaths between 2018 and 2021. Their findings show that deaths during pregnancy as well as the first-year postpartum increased substantially overall during the COVID-19 pandemic. Importantly, their findings put a spotlight on the widening of racial/ethnic inequities in pregnancy-associated mortality from, not only obstetric causes but also substance use, homicide, suicide, and other causes.

SAFEGUARDING HEALTH DURING PREGNANCY

The reality is that the vast majority of pregnancy-associated deaths occurring in the United States can be prevented with timely and equitable access to appropriate, comprehensive, and respectful care. A commitment to doing so requires policies that support person-, family-, and community-based models of prenatal and postnatal care that are also well suited to addressing the social determinants of health and well-being during pregnancy. The COVID-19 pandemic offered a window for exploring expanding access to a broader range of comprehensive care, including birthing centers and the midwifery model of care, doula care, and home birthing.[7] In light of these experiences, in 2023 New York State expanded a pilot program of Medicaid coverage for doula care[8] as well as increased reimbursements for doulas (https://bit.ly/4d6N8lh). Doula care is a community health worker model in which trained, nonmedical coaches provide ongoing and multimodal support before, during, and after childbirth. Multisectoral collaborations, such as the Merck for Mothers program (https://www.merckformothers.com), offer additional examples of partnerships and initiatives directed at reducing pregnancy-associated mortality overall and eliminating racial/ethnic inequities in pregnancy-associated mortality.

By listening to and learning from the stories of people's pregnancy experiences and investing in community-based organizations that support local programs that help make pregnancy safer, we have the answers and the ability to reverse the trends in pregnancy-associated deaths. AJPH

CORRESPONDENCE

Correspondence should be sent to Farzana Kapadia, PhD, MPH, Department of Epidemiology, New York University School of Global Public Health, 708 Broadway, Room 729, New York, NY 10003 (e-mail: farzana.kapadia@nyu.edu). Reprints can be ordered at http://www.ajph.org by clicking the "Reprints" link.

PUBLICATION INFORMATION

Full Citation: Kapadia F. Safeguarding the health of mothers: a public health of consequence, July 2024. *Am J Public Health*. 2024;114(7):672–673.

Acceptance Date: April 24, 2024.

DOI: https://doi.org/10.2105/AJPH.2024.307716

ORCID iD:
Farzana Kapadia https://orcid.org/0000-0003-3459-767X

CONFLICTS OF INTEREST

The author has no conflicts of interest to disclose.

REFERENCES

1. Rossen LM, Womack LS, Hoyert DL, Anderson RN, Uddin SFG. The impact of the pregnancy checkbox and misclassification on maternal mortality trends in the United States, 1999–2017. *Vital Health Stat 3*. 2020;(44):1–61.
2. Hoyert DL, Uddin SFG, Miniño AM. Evaluation of the pregnancy status checkbox on the identification of maternal deaths. *Natl Vital Stat Rep*. 2020;69(1):1–25.
3. Zephyrin LC. Changing the narrative and accelerating action to reduce racial inequities in maternal mortality. *Am J Public Health*. 2021;111(9):1575–1577. https://doi.org/10.2105/AJPH.2021.306462
4. Kumar NR, Borders A, Simon MA. Postpartum Medicaid extension to address racial inequity in maternal mortality. *Am J Public Health*. 2021;111(2):202–204. https://doi.org/10.2105/AJPH.2020.306060
5. Vilda D, Wallace ME, Daniel C, Evans MG, Stoecker C, Theall KP. State abortion policies and maternal death in the United States, 2015–2018. *Am J Public Health*. 2021;111(9):1696–1704. https://doi.org/10.2105/AJPH.2021.306396
6. Centers for Disease Control and Prevention. Update: characteristics of symptomatic women of reproductive age with laboratory-confirmed SARS-CoV-2 infection by pregnancy status—United States, January 22–October 3, 2020. *MMWR Morb Mortal Wkly Rep*. 2020;69(44):1641–1647. https://doi.org/10.15585/mmwr.mm6944e3
7. Profit J, Edmonds BT, Shah N, Cheyney M. The COVID-19 pandemic as a catalyst for more integrated maternity care. *Am J Public Health*. 2020;110(11):1663–1665. https://doi.org/10.2105/AJPH.2020.305935
8. Mehra R, Cunningham SD, Lewis JB, Thomas JL, Ickovics JR. Recommendations for the pilot expansion of Medicaid coverage for doulas in New York State. *Am J Public Health*. 2019;109(2):217–219. https://doi.org/10.2105/AJPH.2018.304797

100 Years of APHA's Public Health Education and Health Promotion Section: Honoring the Legacy of Evart G. Routzahn

Melissa Alperin, EdD, MPH, M. Elaine Auld, MPH, Angela Mickalide, PhD, Regina A. Galer-Unti, PhD, and Marian Moser Jones, PhD, MPH

ABOUT THE AUTHORS

Melissa Alperin is with the Rollins School of Public Health, Emory University, Atlanta, GA. M. Elaine Auld is with the Society for Public Health Education, Washington, DC. Angela Mickalide is a public health education consultant, Edgewater, MD. Regina A. Galer-Unti is an author residing in Urbana, IL. Marian Moser Jones is with the College of Public Health, The Ohio State University, Columbus.

AJPH July 2024, Vol. 114, No. 7

By 1920, the United States was awash in disease prevention messages and materials that were aimed at mass audiences. Over the previous three decades, advances in lithography, colorization, and large-scale mechanized printing had made posters, placards, and postcards available as communication tools. Later in the decade, radio began to be used as a health information medium. Additionally, the new microbial science–based public health leaders used these media to communicate an urgent message of individual responsibility for preventing transmission of infectious agents. During the 1918–1919 influenza pandemic, for example, the US Public Health Service (USPHS) and the American Red Cross produced and distributed millions of color pamphlets and placards in many languages on how to prevent the spread of "flu," some of which featured catchy phrases such as "Cover up each cough and sneeze. If you don't you'll spread disease."[1(p170)] These informational campaigns often featured widely attended public exhibits and lectures. The invention of motion pictures provided an additional, powerful medium for health messaging, with 15 000 movie theaters operating in the United States by 1919 and weekly theater attendance approaching 50 million by 1920.[2,3]

The US government and the American Social Hygiene Association seized on these new media during World War I and launched a massive campaign seeking to prevent sexually transmitted infections (STIs; then called "venereal diseases") among troops and communities near training camps. The program used vivid color posters, pamphlets, illustrated lectures, and films and emphasized sexual abstinence (keeping "clean") as a patriotic obligation. Despite these efforts, STIs became the second most common reason for disability and absences from duty among the armed forces during the war.[4] Then, as now, having an accurate health message did not guarantee success in reception of the message or in producing the sought-after behavior changes. For example, USPHS-produced wartime STI prevention films became popular movie attractions even after the war because of their titillating content, and not necessarily because of their message.[5]

Enter Evart Grant Routzahn. Beginning in 1906, Routzahn directed exhibitions at the National Tuberculosis Association. He then moved to a similar role at the Russell Sage Foundation. Over this period, he studied and refined methods to improve the success of health information materials. In the wake of the war and the pandemic, others in the nascent health education area recognized the need for organization and systematic study of these efforts. In 1921, Routzahn, along with leaders such as Lee Frankel, H. E. Kleinschmidt, William Snow, and Burt Rickards, organized and formed the Health Education and Publicity Section of the American Public Health Association (APHA) and, in doing so, formalized the field in public health.[6]

We discuss Routzahn's and the Public Health Education and Health Promotion (PHEHP) section's intertwined role in developing, systematizing, and disseminating public health education and communication methods. We seek to demonstrate their lasting influence on organized public health on this 100th anniversary of the section's founding.

EVART G. ROUTZAHN

Routzahn was born in Dayton, Ohio, in 1869 and "was educated in the public schools there"[7(p665)] according to his

1939 obituary in *AJPH*. He became a social worker first at the Dayton YMCA and then in Chicago, Illinois. He typified Progressive Era professional reformers, who promoted new scientific, rational approaches to solving social ills. Although a previous generation of social crusaders, many driven by religious convictions, had founded a slew of voluntary organizations to address the growing problems of poverty and disease in the United States' burgeoning but unregulated industrial and commercial centers, this new, more secular, and formally educated generation sought to rationalize, organize, and professionalize these activities.[8]

By the early 1900s, the Progressive ethos began to be infused into public health departments and voluntary public health organizations.[9] The science of germ theory gave public health work precise new tools for diagnosing disease but offered few treatments. In 1882, Robert Koch discovered the causative agent—*Mycobacterium tuberculosis*—for tuberculosis (TB), the leading cause of death among adults. A tuberculin skin test soon made TB easy to diagnose, but the disease continued to flourish in crowded tenement districts. Although some reformers prioritized housing reform and better wages, public health leaders increasingly favored public education as a strategy for reducing the spread of TB.

In 1906, the National Tuberculosis Association hired Routzahn as its first paid employee. Routzahn, known at the YMCA for his "flair for visual expression," was brought on to oversee a touring exhibition designed to bring the message of TB prevention and treatment to the forefront of public concern. Routzahn designed the 50 000 square-foot exhibition with "something to get people to look at, something to explain what people are looking at, and something to get people to talk after they have looked."[10(p42)] It included a "model of an unventilated tuberculosis-breeding bedroom" that exhibition goers could walk through and detailed charts, graphs, and pictures showing how TB spread. When the exhibition toured New York City, Routzahn disseminated print publicity in many languages to tenement neighborhoods, and attendance during its six-week run reached 750 000 people.[10] During this period, he also began to develop methods for analyzing the effectiveness of printed health communication materials, while experimenting with new techniques and media to advance the cause of TB prevention.

In 1912, Routzahn moved to the Russell Sage Foundation, where he served as associate director of the Department of Surveys and Exhibits until his retirement in 1934. In 1913, Mary B. Swain of the Juvenile Protective Association of Chicago asked Routzahn for expert assistance with the *Cycle of Child Life*, an exhibition she was organizing on child health and development.[10] The two, who soon married, went on to jointly develop exhibitions, pamphlets, and other materials.

In 1918, the Routzahns coauthored *The ABC of Exhibit Planning*, a Russell Sage Foundation–published manual that provided a template for developing accurate, meaningful exhibitions and outlined principles of good design that could be applied to other printed health materials.[11] In this volume, the Routzahns cautioned that exhibitors should not become too caught up in the particulars related to which materials should be used, the shipping method, and "how much can be crowded into a given space."[11(p2)] Instead, the focus should be on defining and finding the audience and selecting appropriate facts and methods to gain and hold the attention of the participants.[11] Although the Routzahns' influence is not always recognized, this principle of starting "where the people are" remains a hallmark of the profession of health education more than a century later.

In another piece, Routzahn amplified the importance of designing materials with the intent to reach the audience by citing the work of W. W. Peter, MD, a medical missionary in China. Peter, with his wife Eleanor Whipple Peter, led public health campaigns against smallpox and cholera. Routzahn noted how Peter communicated disease prevention in a way that "gets it across" to the audience. He "gets attention for it; makes it intelligible and interesting to persons unfamiliar with the subject; puts it up in packages that are conveniently carried in the memory and, most important of all, gets it into use."[12(p3)] Additionally, Routzahn noted that Peter employed local people to carry the health message to their communities. These approaches of connecting with an audience through memorable props or devices and through engaging local people as trusted communicators soon became foundational to health educators' work. To this day, community organizing and inclusion of the audience in program planning serve as key strategies for communicating health education and promotion messages.

ORGANIZING HEALTH EDUCATION PROFESSIONALS

In the early 1920s, Routzahn recognized the need to more effectively reach the public via systematic health communication and moved to formally organize a distinct APHA section devoted to public health education. Over the previous years, nationwide support for this field had grown. Following the wartime STI prevention campaigns, the USPHS had begun to recognize the need for organized study and critique of educational strategy, as it produced health materials on many subjects.[13] Health education units began emerging at local and state governmental levels. Meanwhile, at the APHA, organization of the field gained support from Lee K. Frankel, who as vice-president of Metropolitan Life Insurance had in the 1910s penned popular pamphlets on the prevention of TB and other diseases that were distributed by its 14 000 insurance agents.[14] Frankel, who had served as APHA president in 1919, was joined by William F. Snow, leader of the American Social Hygiene Association. Snow also saw a need to improve the science and framework of an emerging profession. In 1921, Frankel and Snow used their national stature and influence to advocate the creation of a new APHA section devoted to public health education and publicity.[13] (Although the section was granted provisional status in 1921 and 1922, with official recognition in 1923,[13,15] the APHA recognizes 1922 as the section's founding year.)

These efforts came to fruition at the 1923 APHA annual meeting. There, Routzahn[13,15] played an instrumental role in gaining official acceptance for a new, full-status Health Education and Publicity section. After securing approval for the section from the APHA Governing Council,[6,7] Routzahn went on to serve as vice-chair, chair, and secretary of the section. The fledgling section aimed to increase the visibility of the field in the APHA and to encourage the professionalization of health education.[6] Underlying these two aims was the belief that health education could and would become central to improving the health of the citizenry.

In 1923, Routzahn began publishing a monthly column—Health Education and Publicity—in *AJPH*. Drawing on the collective wisdom from the Health Education and Publicity section members and other practitioners across the country, Routzahn's compendium of topics included announcements of recently published health department materials, books, upcoming conferences, health articles in the popular literature, health contests, and descriptions of advocacy work. In his columns, he penned practical advice and suggestions for producing effective health education materials and engaging schools and communities, championed innovative ideas, and lent his enthusiasm for health education. For example, in his March 1939 column, he wondered whether health educators had viewed the recent death of Mary Mallon ("Typhoid Mary") as an opportunity to craft local editorials heralding the importance of education and advancing infectious disease controls.[16]

In 1927, section leaders successfully advocated to change the section's name to the Health Education section as the field adopted more systematic health education approaches. At that time, few professional preparation programs in universities or schools of public health offered such instruction. At the APHA annual meetings, the section began to evince its expertise in communication techniques by departing from the staid scientific conference tradition of oral presentations and instead held lively clinics where participants discussed outlines of publicity and education methods and materials. These outlines, submitted by members in advance, covered programs on "diphtheria immunization, attendance at a clinic, vacation precautions, etc."[17(p1191)]

Ahead of the 1928 APHA annual meeting, Routzahn sent section members detailed instructions for the sessions specifying that outlines include the approach employed and materials being used; psychological aspects, such as the presenter's beliefs about the intended audience's "attitude toward" and "level of understanding" about the subject; and "what motives, such as fear, the desire for good looks, civic pride, etc., will be appealed to in seeking action?"[17(p1191)] In this way he reflected the increasing influence of advertising techniques in the field. Overall, these demanding instructions demonstrate how Routzahn, through the section, promoted a systematic and scientifically imbued approach to producing health communications materials.

During Routzahn's tenure, the section's sessions at APHA annual meetings involved lively discussions and demonstrations. Section leaders invited nonmembers to enter the meeting and participate in explanations of advertising, printing, and publicity techniques.[13,15] The innovative "clinic" approach became popular and was used to engage nonmembers and audience members in robust discussions of current problems in health education and public health.

As the section grew and matured, members devoted increased attention to promoting the scientific accuracy of health education messages and adapting them to each audience.[6] The section also initiated a series of multiday health education institutes, held in conjunction with APHA annual meetings and focused on skills building and the application of health education theory or viewpoints of practice. Over the nine years the section conducted these sessions (1933–1942), attendance grew from 25 to 466 participants.[6]

Regrettably, during this era some section members embraced eugenics. In 1934, Peter and section leader Homer Calver brought a German-curated traveling exhibition, *Eugenics in New Germany*, to US cities. It included posters promoting sterilization of the "unfit."[18] This episode shows how health exhibitions—like other mass media—could be misused for nefarious purposes.

Although Routzahn died in 1939, the activities of APHA's Health Education section—renamed the Public Health Education and Health Promotion section in 1990—continued to reflect his influence. He and others in the founding generation presciently understood that health education must keep up with the most popular forms of communication and new media and that it is incumbent on professionals to ensure that the material is accurate, acceptable, and relevant.

The PHEHP section has grown significantly since the early days of pamphlet, poster, and brochure evaluation, yet the principles of appropriate design (enumerated by Routzahn) are still in use today—albeit at a more finely honed theoretical level and with new media having been invented and embraced. The interest stirred by Routzahn and his contemporaries in studying how best to use movies to reach large numbers of people with health information, and in health education to advance behavior change, also have continued through the section's ongoing work.[6] In 1990, the section initiated its first annual public health materials contest. It has since grown in popularity and is still in operation.[19] In the early 2000s, the Health Communications Working Group (a subsection of PHEHP formed in 1997) established the very popular film festival[20] that now attracts a large audience at the APHA annual meeting.

CONCLUSIONS

Anniversaries present an opportunity to reflect, take stock, and prepare for the future, and the authors do so here, as the PHEHP section celebrated its 100-year anniversary in 2022. Over the past century, the PHEHP section has grown to become an integral part of the APHA as documented in the section's digital timeline.[19–22]

As we consider the foundation built by Routzahn and the many health educators who have worked to form and nurture the discipline, we are mindful of the challenges ahead. Routzahn, writing in *AJPH* in 1926, asked, "Are we leading people to believe in us so that they will seek to understand our message and believe that our facts *are* facts?"[23(p336)] In the current era, marked by the spread of deleterious "scientific" misinformation and disinformation, Routzahn would have challenged us to accelerate our quest for effective communication methods and materials. We note that 100 years ago health educators grappled with similar problems. Certainly, the challenges of today's media labyrinth complicate our messaging in ways that Routzahn could never have imagined. Yet, his spirit and dedication inspire PHEHP section members to boldly address the challenges and enigmas of health communications for the next 100 years. AJPH

CORRESPONDENCE

Correspondence should be sent to Melissa Alperin, EdD, MPH, MCHES, Rollins School of Public Health, Emory University, 1518 Clifton Rd, Atlanta, GA 30322 (e-mail: moose.alperin@emory.edu). Reprints can be ordered at http://www.ajph.org by clicking the "Reprints" link.

PUBLICATION INFORMATION

Full Citation: Alperin M, Auld ME, Mickalide A, Galer-Unti RA, Jones MM. 100 years of APHA's Public Health Education and Health Promotion section: honoring the legacy of Evart G. Routzahn. *Am J Public Health*. 2024;114(7):674–678.

Acceptance Date: March 10, 2024.

DOI: https://doi.org/10.2105/AJPH.2024.307663

CONTRIBUTORS

Each author researched the history of Evart Routzahn or the Public Health Education and Health Promotion (PHEHP) section, wrote or heavily edited sections of the article, and approved the final version.

ACKNOWLEDGMENTS

The authors wish to thank Wendy Shay, American Public Health Association archivist; the PHEHP history workgroup; and PHEHP leadership and membership—past, present, and future.

CONFLICTS OF INTEREST

The authors have no conflicts of interest to declare.

REFERENCES

1. Jones MM. *The American Red Cross From Clara Barton to the New Deal*. Baltimore, MD: Johns Hopkins University Press; 2013. https://doi.org/10.1353/book.21077
2. Koszarski R. *An Evening's Entertainment: The Age of the Silent Feature Picture, 1915–1928*. Berkeley, CA: University of California Press; 1990.
3. Kyvig DE. *Daily Life in the United States: Decades of Promise and Pain*. Westport, CT: Greenwood Press; 2001.
4. Siler JF. *The Medical Department of the United States Army in the World War*. Vol. 9: *Communicable and Other Diseases*. Washington, DC: Government Printing Office; 1928.
5. Lord AM. *Condom Nation: The US Government's Sex Education Campaign From World War I to the Internet*. Baltimore, MD: Johns Hopkins University Press; 2010. https://doi.org/10.1353/book.3453
6. Rugen ME. *A Fifty Year History of the Public Health Education Section of the American Public Health Association 1922–1972*. Washington, DC: American Public Health Association; 1972.
7. Evart Grant Routzahn. *Am J Public Health*. 1939; 29(6):665–666. https://doi.org/10.2105/AJPH.29.6.665
8. McGerr M. *A Fierce Discontent: The Rise and Fall of the Progressive Movement in America, 1870–1920*. New York, NY: Oxford University Press; 2005.
9. Duffy J. *The Sanitarians: A History of American Public Health*. Champaign, IL: University of Illinois Press; 1990.
10. Koslow JL. *Exhibiting Health: Public Health Displays in the Progressive Era*. New Brunswick, NJ: Rutgers

University Press; 2020. https://doi.org/10.36019/9781978803305

11. Routzahn EG, Routzahn MS. *The ABC of Exhibit Planning*. New York, NY: The Russell Sage Foundation; 1918.
12. Routzahn EG. *The Health Show Comes to Town*. New York, NY: Russell Sage Foundation; 1920.
13. Kleinschmidt HE. The birth of a section. *Am J Public Health*. 1948;38(12):1657–1662. https://doi.org/10.2105/AJPH.38.12.1657
14. Fee E. Lee K. Frankel (1867–1931): public leader and life insurance executive. *Am J Public Health*. 2011;101(10):1870. https://doi.org/10.2105/AJPH.2009.191072
15. Kleinschmidt HE. Early days of the Public Health Education section. *Am J Public Health*. 1944;34(10):1058–1064. https://doi.org/10.2105/AJPH.34.10.1058
16. Routzahn EG. Public health education. *Am J Public Health*. 1939;29(3):276–281. https://doi.org/10.2105/AJPH.29.3.276
17. Routzahn EG. Education and publicity. *Am J Public Health*. 1928;18(9):1191–1194. https://doi.org/10.2105/AJPH.18.9.1191
18. Rydell R, Cogdell C, Largent M. The Nazi eugenics exhibit in the United States, 1934–43. In: Currell S, Cogdell C, eds. *Popular Eugenics: National Efficiency and American Mass Culture in the 1930s*. Athens, OH: Ohio University Press; 2006: 359–379.
19. Auld ME, Galer-Unti RA, Alperin M, Mickalide A. 100 years of the American Public Health Association's Public Health Education and Health Promotion section: celebrating the past, forging the future. *Health Promot Pract*. [Epub ahead of print March 18, 2024]. https://doi.org/10.1177/15248399241235925
20. McGill N. APHA film festival celebrates 10th anniversary in November: designer Norma Kamali among speakers. *Nation's Health*. 2013;43(8):3.
21. Nicolaus T. PHEHP section marks 100 years of public health education, promotion. *Nation's Health*. 2022;52(8):11.
22. American Public Health Association. Public Health Education and Health Promotion section. PHEHP digital timeline. Available at: https://www.apha.org/APHA-Communities/Member-Sections/Public-Health-Education-and-Health-Promotion/News-and-Events. Accessed February 12, 2023.
23. Routzahn EG. Education and publicity: good news suppressed. *Am J Public Health (N Y)*. 1926;16(3):335–338. https://doi.org/10.2105/AJPH.16.3.335

Addressing Misinformation: A More Nuanced Understanding for Public Health Professionals

Randy Wykoff, MD, MPH&TM, David Harker, PhD, and Leah Loveday

ABOUT THE AUTHORS

Randy Wykoff and Leah Loveday are with the College of Public Health, East Tennessee State University, Johnson City. David Harker is with the College of Arts and Sciences, East Tennessee State University.

The concept of misinformation is understandably receiving a great deal of attention. Recent calls from the US Surgeon General,[1] the World Health Organization,[2] and the American Medical Association,[3] among many others, have all emphasized the importance of health professionals recognizing and speaking out in the face of health misinformation.

The urgency has arisen, at least in part, from the extensive amount of misinformation that has spread relating to COVID-19[4] and the risks of childhood vaccines,[5] but similar problems can be traced back to the tobacco industry's efforts during the second half of the 20th century to sow doubt about the connection between cigarettes and lung cancer[6,7] and, certainly, well beyond that.

The increased amount of misinformation and the growing awareness of its impact on the public's health have led to calls for public health workers and other health professionals to respond to, counter, or correct misinformation to the greatest extent possible.[8]

For health professionals to effectively address misinformation, however, they need to start with an understanding that there are several different ways by which members of the public can be misled, each potentially requiring a different approach on the part of the health professional.

VARIATIONS OF MISINFORMATION

Briefly, we believe that there are at least six variations of misinformation that may require different responses from health professionals.

Intentional Misinformation

Also known as "disinformation," intentional misinformation is characterized by a statement that is made, or a product that is promoted, with the clear knowledge on the part of the speaker or promoter that the information is false. The essential feature of intentional misinformation is the originator's intent to deceive the audience for the purpose of financial or other gain on their part. In the latter part of the 20th century, for example, it became clear from internal documents that there were individuals in the tobacco industry who were aware of the health risks of their products while they continued to publicly deny those risks.[7]

There are other, more current examples of people promoting modern "miracle cures."[9–11] While it may be difficult to dissuade someone from believing intentional misinformation, it may be helpful to draw attention to the profits that the source of such misinformation stands to gain.

Conspiracy-Based Misinformation

Conspiracy-based misinformation results in someone believing that a significant conspiracy both exists and justifies a belief or action that would not otherwise be accepted by the mainstream. The idea that Bill Gates and others were conspiring to introduce microchips into unsuspecting people by use of the COVID-19 vaccine, for example, resulted in people declining to take a potentially life-saving vaccine.[12,13]

Conspiracy-based misinformation may be particularly difficult to counter because those who believe this information have often also rejected the authority of genuinely reliable sources of good information. Furthermore, the health professional attempting to address this misinformation may be seen as a part of (or at least sympathetic to) the "conspiracy."

Intuitive Misinformation

Intuitive misinformation is something that is believed because there is, to at least some extent, some "logic" to the belief. For example, the temporal relationship between the receipt of vaccines with the diagnosis of autism in children has likely influenced those who believe that vaccines "cause" autism, despite overwhelming evidence to the contrary.[14] The distrust of vaccines can be enhanced by other examples of intuitive misinformation. Because people think it is morally worse to harm others by doing something rather than not doing something, parents are more concerned about the negative consequences of vaccinating their children (short-term pain, crying, and longer-term risks of possible side effects) than the risks of not having them vaccinated.[15]

Identity-Based Misinformation

Identity-based misinformation describes situations in which someone has accepted misinformation because that belief is extremely prevalent within (or even required by) one or more of their social, political, or religious affiliations. This can include faith traditions that see a net "negative" in blood transfusions,[16] accessing mental health services,[17] vaccinations,[18] or other accepted medical practices. These beliefs may also hold that a nonmedical intervention, such as prayer or laying-on-hands, is a preferable course of action or even one "required" by their faith. In the case of political affiliations, individuals may choose to follow the guidance and recommendations of political leaders whose interpretation of medical information may differ from the mainstream.[19] People who hold identity-based misinformation may find it difficult to disavow certain beliefs for fear of being ostracized from their peer group.[20] It may also be difficult to disavow these beliefs because of the discomfort of self-contradiction.[21]

Normalized Misinformation

Certain beliefs are so commonly held as to almost be considered cultural norms. The widespread belief that vitamins and dietary supplements are uniformly beneficial for people without underlying nutritional deficiencies is a good example of normalized misinformation. It is so widely held as to be practically unchallengeable, despite the absence of strong supportive scientific evidence.[22] The more widespread a belief is, the more difficult it may be to counter it, especially when there are many health professionals who support the belief, as is the case with multivitamins.[23]

Recent Misinformation

Recent misinformation reflects the situation in which "scientific consensus" and "best available evidence," has only recently changed. The changing recommendations regarding low-dose aspirin for men at low risk of heart disease[24] or the use of hormone-replacement therapy for menopausal women[25] are both examples of situations in which further clinical studies have led to a change in the scientific consensus. Even when the standard of care has changed and the scientific consensus is unambiguous, the public may be unaware of, or unconvinced by, the new consensus. It is also worth noting that while a change in "best available evidence" may necessitate changes in practice or policy, these can have a negative effect on the credibility of the speaker. The public might perceive changes in advice and policy as evidence that relevant experts are not trustworthy or knowledgeable.

This list is not intended to be comprehensive. It is, however, intended to help the health professional understand that people believe inaccurate information for many different reasons and that these reasons may require quite different approaches.

These categories are not, of course, mutually exclusive. Conspiracies can be promoted and stoked intentionally and for the purpose of generating profits. Misinformation can be intuitively appealing, but the associated beliefs can also become part of an individual's sense of identity, and can again be championed by individuals intentionally for selfish ends. As any piece of misinformation becomes more widely accepted within society, it will become more difficult to correct.

THE ROLE OF THE HEALTH PROFESSIONAL

As the health professional considers how best to address a particular piece of misinformation, it is, of course, also worth asking the question "How dangerous is this misinformation?" While it may be intellectually and ethically uncomfortable for the provider to leave any misinformation unchallenged, there are certainly times when it may be worth considering, provided that the health professional is not, then, perceived as supporting or reinforcing that misinformation.

When there is, however, a clear risk to the individual or his family, or when the individual is in a position to further propagate misinformation, it is important for the health professional to address and try to correct the misinformation. To that end, understanding more about the nature of the misinformation, as explored earlier, can be helpful.

Similarly, health professionals should familiarize themselves with studies on the reasons that individuals are more or less susceptible to misinformation[26] and the efficacy of distinct approaches for diminishing its impact,[27] although that is beyond the scope of this editorial.

Because misinformation may have evolved from multiple different sources, as outlined previously, when exposed to a patient or a group that holds an erroneous belief, the health professional should first attempt to understand the origin of that belief. Understanding why someone believes a piece of misinformation may help the health professionals to more effectively correct that misinformation. AJPH

CORRESPONDENCE

Correspondence should be sent to Randy Wykoff, Dean, College of Public Health, PO Box 70623, East Tennessee State University, Johnson City, TN 37614 (e-mail: wykoff@etsu.edu). Reprints can be ordered at https://ajph.org by clicking the "Reprints" link.

PUBLICATION INFORMATION

Full Citation: Wykoff R, Harker D, Loveday L. Addressing misinformation: a more nuanced understanding for public health professionals. *Am J Public Health*. 2024;114(7):679–681.

Acceptance Date: April 5, 2024.

DOI: https://doi.org/10.2105/AJPH.2024.307690

CONTRIBUTORS

L. Loveday conducted significant background research on this topic, including the identification and review of other works in the field. L. Loveday and R. Wykoff crafted the preliminary draft of the article, the latter basing his contributions on a presentation that he had made and on his own work on this topic. D. Harker further modified the initial draft, updating it to reflect his previous work and publications on this topic. All three authors reviewed and edited each draft of the article.

ACKNOWLEDGMENTS

The authors would like to thank and acknowledge their professional colleagues, both at East Tennessee State University and elsewhere, for their work on this important, sensitive, and evolving topic.

CONFLICTS OF INTEREST

The authors report no conflicts of interest.

REFERENCES

1. Murthy V. Confronting health misinformation: the US Surgeon General's advisory on building a healthy information environment. US Department of Health and Human Services. March 7, 2022. Available at: https://www.hhs.gov/sites/default/files/surgeon-general-misinformation-advisory.pdf. Accessed March 26, 2024.
2. World Health Organization. Managing the COVID-19 infodemic: promoting healthy behaviors and mitigating the harm from misinformation and disinformation. Joint statement by WHO, UN, UNICEF, UNDP, UNESCO, UNAIDS, ITU, UN Global Pulse, IFRC. 2020. Available at: https://www.who.int/news/item/23-09-2020-managing-the-covid-19-infodemic-promoting-healthy-behaviours-and-mitigating-the-harm-from-misinformation-and-disinformation. Accessed September 14, 2023.
3. American Medical Association. The AMA adopts new policy aimed at addressing public health disinformation. 2021. Available at: https://www.ama-assn.org/press-center/press-releases/ama-adopts-new-policy-aimed-addressing-public-health-disinformation. Accessed September 14, 2023.
4. Joseph AM, Fernandez V, Kritzman S, et al. COVID-19 misinformation on social media: a scoping review. *Cureus*. 2022;14(4):e24601. https://doi.org/10.7759/cureus.24601.
5. Knudsen J, Perlman-Gabel M, Uccelli IG, Jeavons J, Chokshi DA. Combating misinformation as a core function of public health. *NEJM Catal Innov Care Deliv*. 2023;4(2). https://doi.org/10.1056/CAT.22.0198
6. Oreskes N, Conway E. *Merchants of Doubt: How a Handful of Scientists Obscured the Truth on Issues From Tobacco Smoke to Global Warming*. New York, NY: Bloomsbury Publishing USA; 2011.
7. Brandt A. *The Cigarette Century: the Rise, Fall, and Deadly Persistence of the Product that Defined America*. New York, NY: Basic Books; 2007.
8. Wu JT, McCormick J. Why health professionals should speak out against false beliefs on the Internet. *AMA J Ethics*. 2018;20(11):E1052–E1058. https://doi.org/10.1001/amajethics.2018.1052
9. Liester MB. The chlorine dioxide controversy: a deadly poison or a cure for COVID-19? *Int J Med Med Sci*. 2021;13(2):13–21. https://doi.org/10.5897/IJMMS2021.1461
10. Baker SA, Maddox A. From COVID-19 treatment to miracle cure: the role of influencers and public figures in amplifying the hydroxychloroquine and ivermectin conspiracy theories during the pandemic. *M/C Journal*. 2022;25(1). https://doi.org/10.5204/mcj.2872.
11. Sidley P. Miracle AIDS cure hits the South African press. *BMJ*. 1997;314:450. https://doi.org/10.1136/bmj.314.7078.450
12. Islam MS, Kamal AM, Kabir A, et al. COVID-19 vaccine rumors and conspiracy theories: the need for cognitive inoculation against misinformation to improve vaccine adherence. *PLoS One*. 2021;16(5):e0251605. https://doi.org/10.1371/journal.pone.0251605
13. Freeman D, Loe BS, Chadwick A, et al. COVID-19 vaccine hesitancy in the UK: the Oxford coronavirus explanations, attitudes, and narratives survey (Oceans) II. *Psychol Med*. 2022;52(14):3127–3141. https://doi.org/10.1017/S0033291720005188.
14. Davidson M. Vaccination as a cause of autism—myths and controversies. *Dialogues Clin Neurosci*. 2017;19(4):403–407. https://doi.org/10.31887/DCNS.2017.19.4/mdavidson.
15. Miton H, Mercier H. Cognitive obstacles to pro-vaccination beliefs. *Trends Cogn Sci*. 2015;19(11):633–636. https://doi.org/10.1016/j.tics.2015.08.007
16. Gruberg M. Blood transfusions and medical care against religious beliefs. Middle Tennessee State University Free Speech Center. July 31, 2023. Available at: https://firstamendment.mtsu.edu/article/blood-transfusions-and-medical-care-against-religious-beliefs. Accessed March 28, 2024.
17. Ayvaci ER. Religious barriers to mental healthcare. *Am J Psychiatry Resid J*. 2017;11(7):11–13. https://doi.org/10.1176/appi.ajp-rj.2016.110706
18. Vanderbilt University Occupational Health Clinic. Immunizations and religion. Vanderbilt University Medical Center. 2013. Available at: https://www.vumc.org/health-wellness/resource-articles/immunizations-and-religion. Accessed March 26, 2024.
19. Kates J, Tolbert J, Rouw A. The red/blue divide in COVID-19 vaccination continues: an update. Kaiser Family Foundation. January 19, 2022. Available at: https://www.kff.org/policy-watch/the-red-blue-divide-in-covid-19-vaccination-rates-continues-an-update. Accessed March 26, 2024.
20. De Cruz H. Believing to belong: addressing the novice-expert problem in polarized scientific communication. *Soc Epistemology*. 2020;34(5):440–452. https://doi.org/10.1080/02691728.2020.1739778
21. Guenther CL, Alicke M. Self-enhancement and belief perseverance. *J Exp Soc Psychol*. 2008;44(3):706–712. https://doi.org/10.1016/j.jesp.2007.04.010
22. US Preventive Services Task Force. Final recommendation statement. Vitamin, mineral, and multivitamin supplementation to prevent cardiovascular disease and cancer. June 21, 2022. Available at: https://www.uspreventiveservicestaskforce.org/uspstf/recommendation/vitamin-supplementation-to-prevent-cvd-and-cancer-preventive-medication. Accessed March 26, 2024.
23. The Decision Lab. Band wagon effect. Available at: https://thedecisionlab.com/biases/bandwagon-effect. Accessed March 26, 2024.
24. US Preventive Services Task Force. Final recommendation statement. Aspirin use to prevent cardiovascular disease: preventive medication. April 26, 2022. Available at: https://www.uspreventiveservicestaskforce.org/uspstf/recommendation/aspirin-to-prevent-cardiovascular-disease-preventive-medication. Accessed March 26, 2024.
25. US Preventive Services Task Force. Final recommendation statement. Hormone therapy in postmenopausal persons: primary prevention of chronic conditions. November 1, 2022. Available at: https://www.uspreventiveservicestaskforce.org/uspstf/document/RecommendationStatementFinal/menopausal-hormone-therapy-preventive-medication. Accessed March 26, 2024.
26. Nan X, Wang Y, Thier K. Why people believe health misinformation and who are at risk? A systematic review of individual differences in susceptibility to health misinformation. *Soc Sci Med*. 2022;314(1):115398. https://doi.org/10.1016/j.socscimed.2022.115398
27. Roozenbeek J, van der Linden S. How to combat health misinformation: a psychological approach. *Am J Health Promot*. 2022;36(3):569–575. https://doi.org/10.1177/08901171211070958

The Untapped Potential of Precision Health to Improve Heat Resilience for Those Who Need It Most

Aaron S. Bernstein, MD, MPH, Julia R. Malits, MD, MPH, and Gregory A. Wellenius, ScD

ABOUT THE AUTHORS

Aaron S. Bernstein is with Boston Children's Hospital and the Center for Climate, Health and the Global Environment, Harvard T. H. Chan School of Public Health, Boston, MA. Julia R. Malits is with the Departments of Emergency Medicine at Massachusetts General Hospital and Brigham and Women's Hospital, Boston, MA. Gregory A. Wellenius is with the Center for Climate and Health, Boston University School of Public Health, Boston, MA.

AJPH July 2024, Vol. 114, No. 7

Climate change is fueling more severe and frequent extreme heat events that endanger human health. In the past 30 years, extreme heat has claimed more lives than any other extreme weather event in the United States.[1] Plainly, strategies to prevent morbidity and mortality from heat need improvement. Here, we explore the shortcomings of contemporary heat resilience strategies and share a vision to reduce heat-related harm by applying the principles of precision health.

The heat preparedness strategies of today are inadequate, at least in part, because they are built on a foundation of knowledge gleaned from large population samples. What's gleaned from large samples, though, may fail to protect those most at risk from heat who have attributes furthest from population averages. Heat warning systems, for example, are triggered when a metric of heat (typically, the heat index in the United States) is forecast to surpass a given threshold. However, this threshold choice is seldom tied to health outcomes, is only coarsely tailored to specific locations, and rarely accounts for variability in individual heat exposure. In cities, for example, variations in outdoor temperatures can exceed 20°F (–6.7°C) because of differences in heat retention across urban landscapes.[2] This variability raises the prospect that a monitoring station may not sense a threshold, thus failing to activate a heat alert when necessary. Additionally, heat preparedness strategies often distribute scarce resources based on neighborhood-level social determinants of health, including wealth, health care access, and race.[3] However, substantial variability in the social determinants of health relevant to heat risk—such as social isolation, living on the top floor of a residence, and access to air conditioning—leads to variation in heat exposure even within neighborhoods.

THE UNTAPPED ROLE OF PRECISION HEALTH

These blind spots could be addressed by adopting a precision health approach. Such an approach seeks to probe and leverage information specific to an individual or group joined by geography or by shared biomedical or social factors. A precision health approach could thereby enable better allocation of scarce resources to those who need them most, thus delivering better health outcomes. A precision health–driven approach could allow for innovation of new strategies and, where appropriate, be considered in addition to existing public health strategies that are readily achievable.

In the context of extreme heat, the framework of precision health could be applied to improve heat alert systems' capacity to advance public health. For example, precision health would improve heat exposure assessment by joining regional temperature forecasts to local temperature measurements gathered from diverse settings, including residential buildings (e.g., the temperature gradient between the first and top floors of a multistory building), worksites, and athletic venues. It would also account for heat sensitivity through such factors as race, certain chronic health conditions (e.g., cardiovascular disease and diabetes), time-activity patterns, and potentially genomic variability. Organisms—from mustard plants to humans—have genetically influenced responses to heat stress, and polymorphisms in several candidate genes may underlie variation in heat stroke risk.[4] Variability in genes involved in drug metabolism (e.g., CYP2D6) might also explain why, for example, the use of beta blockers and selective serotonin reuptake inhibitors may increase the risk of hospitalization when temperatures rise.[5]

With more nuanced data input, heat alerts could be issued and resources deployed specifically based on the characteristics of individuals and specific populations most sensitive to heat at temperatures lower than would pose risks to the general population. En masse alerts could be reserved for extraordinary heat events, thus avoiding alarm fatigue among the general population for whom a higher temperature threshold is generally needed.

Beyond enabling more targeted heat alerts, precision health strategies may also inform responses to heat events. Cooling centers are a mainstay of cities' heat response globally. However, they are often underutilized, in part because they are difficult to access owing to social isolation and mobility constraints among at-risk individuals. Although cooling centers will likely always be an important part of heat action plans, precision health could emphasize individualized cooling plans as simple as seeking relief in a neighbor's air-conditioned home, designating communal "cooling spaces" within residential buildings for tenants who cannot afford air conditioning, or allotting appropriate break intervals to outdoor workers. These strategies can be further modified to account for differences between urban and rural communities. Temperature forecasts are sufficiently accurate two or more days before a heat event, allowing time to mobilize a more targeted heat response. Such a targeted approach is already being used in 24 Italian cities.[6]

REQUIRED STAKEHOLDERS AND COLLABORATORS

To deliver a precision health–based heat response in the United States, health care providers and systems must serve as important allies of the public health agencies and atmospheric scientists charged with heat preparedness. Health care providers and systems likely have detailed information on heat risk and resilience factors for their patients, such as age, diagnoses, medications, occupation, and, increasingly, social determinants of health, including energy insecurity and access to air conditioning. Public health agencies, health care providers, and community organizations can then collaboratively apply this knowledge to identify and engage at-risk individuals and communities to establish personalized pathways to resilience. This paradigm is being piloted at frontline clinics across the United States.[7]

A precision health–based approach to heat resilience will also require new collaborations between public health agencies and health care providers as well as researchers, funders, and payors. A promising development in the realm of research funding is the National Institutes of Health Climate Change and Health Initiative. Among its first actions was supporting four Alliance for Community Engagement on Climate and Health sites and a research coordinating center. Together, these entities can catalyze the research and translation needed to innovate equitable climate resilience, which helps people to be healthier and health care utilization and costs to fall. Health care payors ought to take note and explore ways to support climate resilience through public sector partnerships.

THE LIMITATIONS OF PRECISION HEALTH

The promise of precision health to mitigate heat risk does come with limitations. First, gathering and processing relevant genetic, health, and environmental data will require time and financial resources and must be done with a clear focus on health equity. This shortcoming warrants particular consideration in low- and middle-income countries, where relevant information flows may be limited. Moreover, precision health has often been construed to value what can be learned from reductionist biology above qualitative and social science. To the extent that this bias exists, it must be countered, because every community has social dynamics that will override any molecular force in shaping the effectiveness of a heat response. Certainly, precision health cannot repair the structural causes of health inequities that underpin the lion's share of heat risk, and initiatives targeted at structural causes are indispensable. Despite these drawbacks, precision health offers unique pathways to deliver more effective and efficient heat resilience.

THE CLIMATE CRISIS DEMANDS URGENT AND BOLD ACTION

The climate crisis has already intensified the threat of heat and other extreme events—such as flooding, hurricanes, wildfires, and drought—to human health. The rising tide of disasters requires urgent actions that innovate, not merely expand, resilience strategies. We are left with no time to spare in realizing the potential of precision health. AJPH

CORRESPONDENCE

Correspondence should be sent to Julia R. Malits, 55 Fruit St, Boston, MA 02114 (e-mail: jmalits@bwh.harvard.edu). Reprints can be ordered at https://www.ajph.org by clicking the "Reprints" link.

PUBLICATION INFORMATION

Full Citation: Bernstein AS, Malits JR, Wellenius GA. The untapped potential of precision health to improve heat resilience for those who need it most. *Am J Public Health*. 2024;114(7):682–684.

Acceptance Date: April 8, 2024.

DOI: https://doi.org/10.2105/AJPH.2024.307688

CONTRIBUTORS

A. S. Bernstein and G. A. Wellenius conceptualized the manuscript. A. S. Bernstein, G. A. Wellenius, and J. R. Malits contributed equally to the writing and editing of the manuscript. J. R. Malits prepared the manuscript for submission.

CONFLICTS OF INTEREST

G. A. Wellenius serves as a consultant for the Health Effects Institute (Boston, MA) and Google LLC (Mountain View, CA) and serves as a co-principal investigator of the BUSPH-HSPH Climate Change and Health Research Coordinating Center (CAFÉ) funded under the National Institutes of Health's Climate Change and Health Initiative (https://www.nih.gov/climateandhealth). A. S. Bernstein has received funding from Biogen (Cambridge, MA) and Johnson and Johnson (New Brunswick, NJ) to support work on climate resilience.

REFERENCES

1. National Weather Service. Weather fatalities 2021. Available at: https://www.weather.gov/hazstat. Accessed May 5, 2023.
2. Mentaschi L, Duveiller G, Zulian G, et al. Global long-term mapping of surface temperature shows intensified intra-city urban heat island extremes. *Glob Environ Change*. 2022;72:102441. https://doi.org/10.1016/j.gloenvcha.2021.102441
3. New York City Dept of Health and Mental Hygiene. Interactive heat vulnerability index. Available at: https://a816-dohbesp.nyc.gov/IndicatorPublic/data-features/hvi/ https://a816-dohbesp.nyc.gov/IndicatorPublic/EPHTPDF/HVI_FAQ.pdf. Accessed December 7, 2022.
4. Bouchama A, Abuyassin B, Lehe C, et al. Classic and exertional heatstroke. *Nat Rev Dis Primers*. 2022;8(1):8. https://doi.org/10.1038/s41572-021-00334-6
5. Kalisch Ellett LM, Pratt NL, Le Blanc VT, Westaway K, Roughead EE. Increased risk of hospital admission for dehydration or heat-related illness after initiation of medicines: a sequence symmetry analysis. *J Clin Pharm Ther*. 2016;41(5):503–507. https://doi.org/10.1111/jcpt.12418
6. Regional Health System. Heat waves: prevention and support for people at risk. Available at: https://www.aslroma1.it/news/ondate-di-calore-prevenzione-e-supporto-alle-persone-a-rischio. Accessed December 14, 2022.
7. Americares. The climate resilience for frontline clinics toolkit. Available at: https://www.americares.org/what-we-do/community-health/climate-resilient-health-clinics. Accessed May 11, 2023.

Listening Sessions to Shape the Innovative NIH ComPASS Common Fund Program to Advance Health Equity

Alison G. M. Brown, PhD, RDN, Danyelle Winchester, PhD, Shalanda A. Bynum, PhD, MPH, Sara M. Amolegbe, MSPH, Yvonne O. Ferguson, PhD, MPH, Minnjuan Flournoy Floyd, PhD, MPH, MBA, Collene Lawhorn, PhD, Jimmy T. Le, ScD, MA, Jacqueline Lloyd, PhD, MSW, April Y. Oh, PhD, MPH, Nadra Tyus, DrPH, MPH, Damiya E. Whitaker, PsyD, MA, and Cheryl Anne Boyce, PhD

The National Institutes of Health (NIH) recognized the need for a research program to address the underlying structural factors that impact health. To inform the development of the NIH Common Fund Community Partnerships to Advance Science for Society (ComPASS) Program, NIH obtained input through community listening sessions. Through its design, ComPASS recognizes the essential role of community organizations as the lead in addressing persistent structural and social challenges to accelerate progress toward advancing health equity. (*Am J Public Health*. 2024;114(7):685–689. https://doi.org/10.2105/AJPH.2024.307656)

AJPH July 2024, Vol. 114, No. 7

To address the structural inequities that impact health and perpetuate health disparities,[1] the National Institutes of Health (NIH) Common Fund launched the innovative, 10-year Community Partnership to Advance Science for Society (ComPASS) research program. The NIH Common Fund supports unique, emerging scientific opportunities and pressing challenges in biomedical research that are of high priority across the many components of NIH.[2] The vision of ComPASS is to support structural intervention research to accelerate progress toward eliminating health disparities and advancing health equity. Structural interventions attempt to change the social, physical, economic, or political environments that may shape or constrain health behaviors and outcomes.[3] They can also address social determinants of health such as economic instability, limited educational and employment opportunities, access to quality housing and healthy food, and lack of community resources.[4]

INTERVENTION AND IMPLEMENTATION

To inform the development of the ComPASS Program, funded by the NIH Common Fund,[2] the ComPASS Working Group, a diverse, interdisciplinary team of scientific staff from across NIH, organized a series of virtual listening sessions. These listening sessions ensured that the program received input from diverse communities, including those historically underserved or underrepresented in research.

PLACE, TIME, AND PERSONS

Between October and November 2021, the ComPASS Working Group convened eight virtual listening sessions and received feedback on research opportunities, challenges, and community needs to address structural and social factors influencing health and perpetuating health disparities. The NIH team conducted broad outreach using social media, e-mail lists, and newsletters from professional societies, community organizations, researchers, and advocacy organizations. There was a high level of interest, resulting in more than 2000 registrants and more than 500 attendees from diverse sectors, including academic organizations, minority-serving and low-resource institutions, community organizations, faith-based institutions, nonprofit organizations, and Tribal communities.

The virtual sessions opened with community leaders reiterating the importance of community voices in research. Facilitated breakout groups encouraged optimal participation and engagement. NIH staff posed open-ended questions about research opportunities, challenges, and needs relevant to health disparities and related interventions. Listening sessions included accessibility options for those with disabilities and limited English proficiency (e.g., sign language interpreting, real-time transcription, and spoken language interpreters for participants with limited English proficiency).

PURPOSE

Listening sessions are valuable tools for obtaining feedback from the research community and health organizations as well as from communities experiencing health disparities. They provide a platform to voice concerns and reveal unique experiences and perspectives and may help improve participation in the research process among racial and ethnic minorities and other historically disenfranchised groups.[5] Their design allows participants to voice opinions and promotes trust on issues such as health equity.[6]

EVALUATION AND ADVERSE EFFECTS

After a review of listening session summaries, subject matter experts synthesized the content, identifying reoccurring themes. Here, we discuss these major themes and key discussion points (Box 1).

Community Ownership

Attendees expressed concerns that the NIH research paradigm places academic research institutions at the forefront of addressing health challenges and has systematically limited community organizations' ownership and contributions to addressing pressing health issues within their communities. This research paradigm has contributed to inequities between the community and the research enterprise by giving research institutions control over community involvement in research, distribution of funding to communities, and prioritization of health topics and solutions. Giving community organizations ownership of the research is one strategy to empower communities in the research process.

Community Capacity Building

Participants expressed the need for capacity building for community organizations and their community-based research partners to effectively develop, implement, and sustain structural health equity interventions. Building capacity within the community fosters sustainable resources to address health challenges and the structural and social factors that affect them. Health research interventions will have a limited, short-term impact without community capacity building and resources for the future.[8]

Community Relationships and Building Trust

Session participants expressed the need for research organizations to build authentic, trusting relationships with communities. Discussions included the need for research organizations to repair trust from past research involvements. Attempts to proactively develop and maintain trust over time cannot ignore the historical trauma (cumulative multigenerational trauma experienced by descendants of a collective group) and "helicopter research" experiences (when researchers conduct studies with historically marginalized groups with little or no involvement from those communities).[9,10] Participants also questioned if the unequal disease burden sometimes leads researchers to take advantage of those desperately seeking better access to treatment and health outcomes. Disingenuous relationships developed solely for research recruitment impede meaningful community connections and erode community trust, which is required for genuine partnerships.[11]

Bidirectional Learning

Participants emphasized the importance of bidirectional learning to contribute to shared knowledge between researchers and the community. Community partners should collectively engage in discussions and share their experiences as part of the research process. Community members' lived experiences and perspectives add substantial value to health equity efforts.[12] The status quo, where researchers' voices are valued more than community voices, contradicts the mission of advancing health equity.

Public–Private Partnerships in Community Health

Participants suggested developing multisectoral partnerships involving government (e.g., local, state, and federal) and private organizations to collectively

BOX 1— Listening Sessions Themes and Key Discussion Points: National Institutes of Health (NIH) Common Fund Community Partnerships to Advance Science for Society (ComPASS) Program

Theme	Key Discussion Points
Community ownership	• The lack of community ownership creates "health equity tourists." This term has been described in the literature and is defined as researchers interested in health disparities because of current trends but who lack experience with and long-term commitment to health equity research and community-engaged work.[7] • Transformation requires genuine partnerships rather than transactional relationships, calling for a shift from community engagement to community ownership. • Current NIH funding mechanisms typically fund biomedical research institutions as the primary institutions on awards. Increasing awards to community organizations as the primary institution will increase power, funding, and equity for community partners.
Community relationships and building trust	• Grant funding seems inflexible. When the funding periods end, communities can become disappointed and reluctant to participate in future research. Long-term allyship and investment can sustain community trust and enable participation in future research. • NIH needs to be more present in communities. Increasing NIH's attention and visibility in communities could increase its acceptability as a true partner in addressing health disparities.
Community capacity building	• Efforts to support community ownership and empowerment must focus on capacity building among community organizations, academic institutions, and other partners. • Capacity building is central to enabling community organizations to pursue funding independently of academic institutions. • Sustainable funding is needed to develop infrastructure for community engagement independent from individual research projects. • Organizations need lead time built into funding mechanisms to develop the capacity of community partners so they are prepared to engage in community work.
Bidirectional learning	• Nationally available training and education in intervention science is needed. The training should be available to researchers, community organizations, and others engaged in research and meet NIH standards on rigor. • There is a need for training that addresses how to engage community partners and create research products that matter to both the community and researchers. • Investing in community education could build awareness and trust in research.
Public–private partnerships in community health	• NIH should consider investments in research partnerships supporting community-led intervention research and facilitating the sustainability of postfunding efforts. • Community organizations should be respected as equal partners. Agreements stipulating how the partnership will function could be established, similar to academic institutions' partnerships with each other. • Community-led research is enhanced through multisectoral partnerships allowing greater consideration of how research findings inform policy.
Navigating the NIH enterprise	• Encourage funding announcements that provide longer turnaround times to enable sufficient time for community partners to be involved in study design (e.g., measurement and data collection strategy development). Funding timelines are incredibly challenging for early career researchers working to establish partnerships with communities. • Funding opportunities can be innovative in communicating and assessing what counts as research contributions. NIH application biosketches can be allowed to reflect the value of experiences in community-engaged research. • NIH can create funding opportunities that encourage or require establishing partnerships with communities or community organizations, emphasizing equity in resource allocation and sharing (e.g., measures to assess equity in partnerships). • Diversifying review panels to include diverse sociodemographic and experiential composition is necessary to advance equity in review and address underrepresentation and broaden participation in funding.

support health equity efforts. Participants recognized advancing health equity requires the involvement of sectors beyond those focused on health care, such as transportation, neighborhood environment, and healthy food access.[7]

Navigating the NIH Enterprise

Community organizations and other resource-limited organizations were noted to be at a disadvantage when applying for and managing NIH funding. Institutions underrepresented in NIH's funded research require assistance in navigating the complexity of the NIH grant system. Community organizations also identified challenges related to funding opportunities, NIH application procedures, and systems. Participants suggested enhanced support and training for new NIH applicants.

Together, these themes informed strategic planning for ComPASS as a community-led research initiative to build structural interventions for health equity.

SUSTAINABILITY

The insightful perspectives gleaned from the listening sessions informed the overall goals and three synergistic initiatives of the 10-year NIH ComPASS Program. The goals of ComPASS are to (1) study ways to address underlying structural factors within communities that affect health to reduce health disparities and (2) develop a new research model for NIH where the projects are led by community organizations, in collaboration with research partners.[13]

ComPASS funds community organizations to plan, develop, implement, and assess community-led, health equity structural interventions (CHESIs). Structural interventions aim to change the social, physical, and economic environments external to the individual and not under their control that may shape or constrain health behaviors and outcomes.[3,14] They also address social determinants of health, which NIH defines as "the conditions in which people are born, grow, learn, work, play, live, and age, and the wider set of structural factors shaping the conditions of daily life."[15] Influenced by structural racism and discrimination, these include economic instability, limited educational and employment opportunities, access to quality housing and healthy food, lack of community resources, and other conditions of daily life. The CHESIs are supported by the ComPASS Coordination Center, which leads overall program management and coordination of administrative, data, capacity-building, partnership, and training, and the Health Equity Research Hubs (Hubs), which provide localized technical assistance and scientific support as well as support for research capacity-building and training.

Building upon the insights from the listening sessions, ComPASS serves as a new health equity research model to stimulate community-led research. For the first time in an NIH-wide initiative, the CHESI opportunity required community organizations to lead the research applications, collaborating with research partners. This is a shift from the traditional investigator-initiated proposal led by a research organization, increasing parity in the research and discovery process for communities. The focus on training and empowering community organizations for independent initiative sustenance is vital for enduring impact and long-term sustainability. It also aligns with other NIH initiatives to stimulate health disparities research valuing community engagement and building trust.[16]

Serving as a model for future NIH efforts, ComPASS intentionally sought to broaden participation and support first-time community organization applicants in navigating the complexities of the NIH research enterprise. The NIH held an unprecedented eight live technical assistance webinars and office hours for applicants and their research partners, reaching more than 2400 participants and receiving more than 3300 views. Efforts to ensure accessibility, inclusivity, and transparency signify our commitment to broad participation and cement the ComPASS's foundation, ensuring its relevance and impact extend well into the future.[17]

Community input about moving beyond traditional health care contexts determined ComPASS requirements for multisectoral collaborations. Multisectoral Health Equity Research Assemblies, including community, public health, government, and policy partners, will inform structural intervention development at both the local community and national levels to enhance program success and sustainability. The listening sessions also emphasized the need for research capacity building and training for community organizations and their research partners. The ComPASS Hubs will provide tailored technical assistance to the intervention projects to meet their specific research needs. The research capacity building and training support will provide bidirectional learning opportunities to communities, research partners, federal agencies, and others. External communication efforts will ensure the dissemination of data, resources, and tools so that knowledge gained through the ComPASS Program is accessible and sustained for broader public health impact.

The ComPASS Working Group plans to monitor the reach, implementation, and impact of the ComPASS model on developing and evaluating structural interventions to address health inequities. This includes informing the public, the scientific community, and the NIH community on successes and lessons learned from the program.

PUBLIC HEALTH SIGNIFICANCE

Community voices and perspectives shaped the ComPASS Program as an innovative model for community engagement. The NIH used key themes and findings from the listening sessions to inform the program development and leverage lessons learned for successful implementation. The integration of community feedback into the development of ComPASS from its inception created the paradigm shift to stimulate community-led research at NIH, transform health equity research, and advance health for all. AJPH

ABOUT THE AUTHORS

Alison G. M. Brown is with the National Heart Lung and Blood Institute, National Institutes of Health (NIH), Bethesda, MD. Danyelle Winchester is with the Office of Science Policy, NIH. Shalanda A. Bynum is with the National Institute of Nursing Research, NIH. Sara M. Amolegbe, Nadra Tyus, and Cheryl Anne Boyce are with the Office of Strategic Coordination—The Common Fund, NIH. Yvonne O. Ferguson was with the Office of Strategic Coordination–The Common Fund, NIH, during the listening sessions and writing of the manuscript. Minnjuan Flournoy Floyd is with the National Institute of Diabetes and Digestive and Kidney Diseases, NIH. Collene Lawhorn is with the National Institute of Mental Health, NIH. Jimmy T. Le is with the National Eye Institute, NIH. Jacqueline Lloyd is with the Office of Disease Prevention, NIH. April Y. Oh is with the National Cancer Institute, NIH. Damiya E. Whitaker is with the National Institute on Alcohol Abuse and Alcoholism, NIH, and was with the Office of Research on Women's Health, NIH, during the listening sessions and writing of the manuscript.

CORRESPONDENCE

Correspondence should be sent to Alison G. M. Brown, 6705 Rockledge Dr, Bethesda, MD 20817 (e-mail: alison.brown@nih.gov). Reprints can be ordered at https://ajph.org by clicking the "Reprints" link.

PUBLICATION INFORMATION

Full Citation: Brown AGM, Winchester D, Bynum SA, et al. Listening sessions to shape the innovative NIH ComPASS Common Fund program to advance health equity. *Am J Public Health*. 2024;114(7):685–689.

Acceptance Date: March 5, 2024.

DOI: https://doi.org/10.2105/AJPH.2024.307656

CONTRIBUTORS

A. G. M. Brown developed the article outline and contributed to the writing and editing of the article. D. Winchester, S. A. Bynum, S. M. Amolegbe, M. Flournoy Floyd, C. Lawhorn, J. T. Le, J. Lloyd, A. Y. Oh, N. Tyus, and D. E. Whitaker provided input on the outline and contributed to the writing and editing of the article. Y. O. Ferguson and C. A. Boyce provided input on the outline and contributed to the editing of the article.

ACKNOWLEDGMENTS

We would first like to thank the attendees of the listening sessions who shared their insights, expertise, and experience to help inform the development of the Community Partnerships to Advance Science for Society (ComPASS) Program. We would also like to thank the community leaders who welcomed the listening session attendees and gave opening remarks: Debra Furr-Holden, E. Yvonne Lewis, Kendrick E. Curry, Elena Rios, Valarie Blue Bird Jernigan, Bobby Saunkeah, Arleen Brown, Mona AuYoung, Richard Lee, and Lauren Supplee. We would like to acknowledge the ComPASS Working Group members who helped to plan and facilitate the listening sessions and the leadership and strategic direction of the ComPASS co-chairs Janine Clayton (director, Office of Research on Women's Health), Joshua Gordon (director, National Institute of Mental Health), Eliseo Perez-Stables (director, National Institute on Minority Health and Health Disparities), and Shannon Zenk (director, National Institute of Nursing Research), and former co-chair Dave Wilson (director, Tribal Health Research Office).

CONFLICTS OF INTEREST

The authors report no conflicts of interest.

HUMAN PARTICIPANT PROTECTION

Human participant protection is not applicable because the listening sessions were not for research purposes and were used to inform the federal program design and development.

REFERENCES

1. National Academies of Sciences, Engineering, and Medicine; Health and Medicine Division; Board on Population Health and Public Health Practice; Baciu A, Negussie Y, Geller A, et al., eds. *Communities in Action: Pathways to Health Equity*. Washington, DC: National Academies Press; 2017.
2. National Institutes of Health Office of Strategic Coordination. About the NIH Common Fund. Available at: https://commonfund.nih.gov. Accessed May 4, 2023.
3. Brown AF, Ma GX, Miranda J, et al. Structural interventions to reduce and eliminate health disparities. *Am J Public Health*. 2019;109(suppl 1):S72–S78. https://doi.org/10.2105/AJPH.2018.304844
4. Office of Disease Prevention and Health Promotion. Social determinants of health. Healthy People 2030. Available at: https://health.gov/healthypeople/priority-areas/social-determinants-health. Accessed May 4, 2023.
5. Cunningham-Erves J, Stewart EC, Duke J, et al. Use of community listening sessions to disseminate research findings to past participants and communities. *J Community Health*. 2022;47(2):201–210. https://doi.org/10.1007/s10900-021-01038-4
6. National Institutes of Health. UNITE external listening sessions: summary report. Available at: https://www.nih.gov/sites/default/files/research-training/initiatives/ending-structural-racism/RFI_UNITE_external-listening-session-summary-report-508%5B42%5D.pdf. Accessed July 17, 2023.
7. Lopez N, Gadsden VL. Health inequities, social determinants, and intersectionality. Discussion paper. *NAM Perspectives*. Washington, DC: National Academy of Medicine; 2016. https://doi.org/10.31478/201612a.
8. Hacker K, Tendulkar SA, Rideout C, et al. Community capacity building and sustainability: outcomes of community-based participatory research. *Prog Community Health Partnersh*. 2012;6(3):349–360. https://doi.org/10.1353/cpr.2012.0048
9. *Nature* addresses helicopter research and ethics dumping. *Nature*. 2022;606(7912):7. https://doi.org/10.1038/d41586-022-01423-6.
10. Sotero M. A conceptual model of historical trauma: implications for public health practice and research. *J Health Dispar Res Pract*. 2006;1(1):93–108. Available at: https://ssrn.com/abstract=1350062. Accessed August 23, 2023.
11. Organizing Committee for Assessing Meaningful Community Engagement in Health & Health Care Programs & Policies. *Assessing Meaningful Community Engagement: A Conceptual Model to Advance Health Equity Through Transformed Systems for Health. NAM Perspectives. Commentary*. Washington, DC: National Academy of Medicine; 2022.
12. Beames JR, Kikas K, O'Gradey-Lee M, et al. A new normal: integrating lived experience into scientific data syntheses. *Front Psychiatry*. 2021;12:763005. https://doi.org/10.3389/fpsyt.2021.763005
13. National Institutes of Health. NIH launches community-led research program to advance health equity. September 27, 2023. Available at: https://www.nih.gov/news-events/news-releases/nih-launches-community-led-research-program-advance-health-equity. Accessed September 27, 2023.
14. Centers for Disease Control and Prevention. Compendium of evidence-based interventions and best practices for HIV prevention. Structural interventions review methods chapter. Available at: https://www.cdc.gov/hiv/pdf/research/interventionresearch/compendium/si/SI_Chapter_Review_Methods.pdf. Accessed August 23, 2023.
15. National Institute of Nursing Research. NIH SDOH Conceptualization. NIH-wide Social Determinants of Health Research Coordinating Committee. Available at: https://www.ninr.nih.gov/researchandfunding/nih-sdohrcc#tabs2. Accessed August 15, 2023.
16. National Institutes of Health. Minority health and health disparities research. Available at: https://www.nih.gov/ending-structural-racism/minority-health-health-disparities-research. Accessed May 16, 2023.
17. General Services Administration. Section 508 of the Rehabilitation Act. Available at: https://www.section508.gov/manage/laws-and-policies/#:~:text=Section%20508%20of%20the%20Rehabilitation,accessible%20to%20people%20with%20disabilities. Accessed July 19, 2023.

Restoring and Expanding Pandemic-Era Support Policies to Reduce Economic Precarity and Overdose Deaths

Alexandria Macmadu, PhD

ABOUT THE AUTHOR

Alexandria Macmadu is with the Department of Epidemiology, Brown University School of Public Health, Providence, RI.

See also Opioids, COVID-19, & Fatal Overdoses, pp. 693–722.

The COVID-19 pandemic wrought significant economic strife and uncertainty. In December 2020, 38% of adults in the United States were struggling to cover usual household expenses, including food, basic utilities, and medical expenses.[1] In the same period, 20% of renters were behind on rent payments, and 14% of households lacked enough food to eat.[1] Fortunately, many of these measures of hardship were attenuated by pandemic relief programs: by April 2021, 27% of adults were struggling to cover household expenses, 15% of renters were behind on payments, and 8% of households lacked enough food to eat.[2] However, economic precarity rapidly resurged with the expiration of pandemic relief programs and was further amplified by inflation. As of February 2024, 36% of US adults reported struggling to cover usual household expenses,[3] representing a near return to midpandemic levels of economic hardship.

As economic precarity has stubbornly persisted, so too has preventable overdose mortality in the United States. Provisional drug overdose death data indicate that from the 12-month period ending in December 2020 to the 12-month period ending in September 2023, overdose mortality increased by 19% to more than 111 000 deaths nationwide.[4] While economic precarity and overdose deaths are tightly linked,[5] emergent research in this issue of *AJPH* has demonstrated that robust economic support policies can effectively alleviate both.

In this issue, Wolf et al. (p. 714) documented that COVID-19–era economic support policies significantly reduced overdose rates at the state level, though these effects were mitigated by co-occurring measures that limited in-person activities and magnified overdose risk. Findings from Wolf et al. reinforce the need to both restore and expand economic support policies that were implemented at the height of the COVID-19 pandemic. Namely, by bolstering employment and incomes and by reducing household debts and expenses, we can achieve the dual benefits of alleviating economic precarity and stemming the rising tide of overdose deaths.

BOLSTERING EMPLOYMENT AND INCOMES

Previous research has documented that both unemployment and lower wages are linked to drug overdose deaths.[6] By implementing policies that increase employment rates and the availability of jobs providing livable wages, state and federal policymakers can bolster net household incomes while meaningfully reducing overdose fatalities. While the national unemployment rate has declined precipitously since the height of the COVID-19 pandemic, the labor force participation rate—which accounts for those who have given up looking for work—is near its lowest level in recent decades. In January 2024, the labor force participation rate reached 62.5%, continuing its trajectory of steady decline since its historic high of 67% in the early 2000s.[7] Persisting low levels of labor force participation underscore the need for continued and strategic investment in job creation beyond the pandemic-era Infrastructure Investment and Jobs Act.

Similarly, since 2009, the US minimum wage has stagnated at the rate of $7.25 per hour. As of January 2024, many jurisdictions have passed state-level minimum wage laws, ranging from $8.75 to $16.28 hourly. However, $7.25 hourly is the prevailing minimum wage in 20 states, which are concentrated across the US South and Midwest. If enacted in 2024, the Raise the Wage Act would raise the federal minimum in annual increments to $17 per hour by 2029. Given that economic precarity is a determinant of overdose death,[6] policies to raise minimum wages have the potential to significantly reduce overdose rates at the state and national levels.

AJPH July 2024, Vol. 114, No. 7

Lastly, increasing and expanding current unemployment insurance (UI) programs is essential to bolster incomes in the face of persisting low labor force participation. The Coronavirus Aid, Relief, and Economic Security Act supplemented UI payments by $600 weekly and lifted millions of people out of poverty before the provision expired in July 2020.[2] After that, the American Rescue Plan Act (ARPA) continued a $300 weekly supplement to UI payments from December 2020 to September 2021. Once this second supplement expired, UI payments returned to insufficient, prepandemic rates thereafter and have since remained unchanged. By resuming pandemic-era investment in UI programs to raise benefit levels and extend benefit durations, and by expanding eligibility criteria for these programs to include additional classes of workers, significant reductions in overdose mortality can also be achieved.

REDUCING HOUSEHOLD DEBTS AND EXPENSES

Pandemic-era economic support policies realized their efficacy in reducing financial precarity by increasing net incomes and by simultaneously reducing household debts and expenses. One key program, the Supplemental Nutrition Assistance Program (SNAP), continued to be one of the most effective programs for reducing economic precarity during the COVID-19 pandemic—bringing 2.8 and 3.7 million people out of poverty in 2021 and 2022, respectively,[8] and effectively reducing household costs spent on sustenance. At the beginning of the pandemic, SNAP benefits were increased nationwide by 15%, and benefit levels were increased to the maximum level previously allowed by household size for all households, but these program enhancements expired in September 2021 and March 2023, respectively. By restoring these previous levels of investment in SNAP and expanding program eligibility, significant reductions in economic precarity can also be restored.

The child tax credit and the earned income tax credit similarly brought an estimated 7.5 million people out of poverty because of expansions made under the ARPA in 2021.[8] The enhanced child tax credit increased the maximum tax credit from $2000 per child, which was partially refundable, to $3000 per child and $3600 per child aged younger than six years, and it was fully refundable. The earned income tax credit, which was expanded for adults without children, roughly tripled the maximum credit to $1502, increased the income limit, and expanded credit eligibility. Enhancements to both programs have expired, along with the economic stability that they provided, but reinstating and expanding these programs could serve to restore the benefits yielded under the ARPA.

Finally, while pandemic-era eviction moratoria provided significant protections for renters, more substantial and more impactful investments can be made to ensure affordable and accessible housing for all. Greater investment in rental assistance programs and Housing First program models[9] and establishing a national Homes Guarantee[10] would also serve to expand access to long-term, stable, and affordable housing—thereby alleviating economic precarity and reducing overdose risk among those who are most vulnerable.

CONCLUSIONS

Now that the highest waves of the COVID-19 pandemic have subsided, along with the need for stringent social distancing measures that exacerbate overdose risk, an opportunity exists for states to fully realize the benefits of economic support policies on both poverty reduction and overdose prevention. Critically, given the substantial economic impact of substance use disorders and overdose mortality on state budgets,[11] robust implementation of economic support policies at the state and federal levels also has the potential to generate net cost savings. Decarceration and divestment from policing[12] could also serve to address root causes of economic precarity, further reduce overdose risk, and lighten local budgets to enhance funding for social safety nets.

While the strategies outlined here are not comprehensive, and other economic support policies and investments—including in harm reduction approaches—will be essential to curb overdose deaths, these recommendations represent a shift to smarter spending and a more holistic approach to addressing the social and structural determinants of health. By restoring, expanding, and, in some cases, surpassing COVID-19–era economic support policies, state and federal policymakers can alleviate economic precarity for millions and prevent countless thousands of overdose fatalities in years to come. AJPH

CORRESPONDENCE

Correspondence should be sent to Alexandria Macmadu, PhD, Department of Epidemiology, Brown University School of Public Health, 121 S Main St, Box G-S-121-2, Providence, RI 02912 (e-mail: alexandria_macmadu@brown.edu). Reprints can be ordered at https://ajph.org by clicking the "Reprints" link.

PUBLICATION INFORMATION

Full Citation: Macmadu A. Restoring and expanding pandemic-era support policies to reduce economic precarity and overdose deaths. *Am J Public Health*. 2024;114(7):690–692.

Acceptance Date: April 17, 2024.

DOI: https://doi.org/10.2105/AJPH.2024.307701

ORCID iD:
Alexandria Macmadu https://orcid.org/0000-0001-7640-2215

ACKNOWLEDGMENTS

The author wishes to express her gratitude to RSG for his many years of encouragement and support and his thoughtful dialogue on this topic.

CONFLICTS OF INTEREST

The author reports no conflicts of interest.

REFERENCES

1. Center on Budget and Policy Priorities. Tracking the COVID-19 economy's effects on food, housing, and employment hardships. 2022. Available at: https://www.cbpp.org/research/poverty-and-inequality/tracking-the-covid-19-recessions-effects-on-food-housing-and. Accessed March 9, 2024.
2. Trisi D. Government's pandemic response turned a would-be poverty surge into a record poverty decline. Center on Budget and Policy Priorities. August 29, 2023. Available at: https://www.cbpp.org/research/poverty-and-inequality/governments-pandemic-response-turned-a-would-be-poverty-surge-into. Accessed March 9, 2024.
3. US Census Bureau. Household Pulse Survey Interactive Tool. 2024. Available at: https://www.census.gov/data-tools/demo/hhp/#/?measures=EXPENSE. Accessed March 9, 2024.
4. Ahmad FB, Cisewski JA, Rossen LM, Sutton P. Provisional drug overdose data. National Center for Health Statistics. 2024. Available at: https://www.cdc.gov/nchs/nvss/vsrr/drug-overdose-data.htm. Accessed March 9, 2024.
5. Altekruse SF, Cosgrove CM, Altekruse WC, Jenkins RA, Blanco C. Socioeconomic risk factors for fatal opioid overdoses in the United States: findings from the Mortality Disparities in American Communities Study (MDAC). *PLoS One*. 2020;15(1):e0227966. https://doi.org/10.1371/journal.pone.0227966
6. Olfson M, Cosgrove C, Altekruse SF, Wall MM, Blanco C. Deaths of despair: adults at high risk for death by suicide, poisoning, or chronic liver disease in the US. *Health Aff (Millwood)*. 2021;40(3):505–512. https://doi.org/10.1377/hlthaff.2020.01573
7. Hayes A. Labor force participation rate: purpose, formula, and trends. 2024. Available at: https://www.investopedia.com/terms/p/participationrate.asp. Accessed March 15, 2024.
8. Ross K. Poverty rose in 2022, but policy solutions can create a more equitable economy. Center for American Progress. 2023. Available at: https://www.americanprogress.org/article/poverty-rose-in-2022-but-policy-solutions-can-create-a-more-equitable-economy. Accessed March 15, 2024.
9. Pollack CE, Saloner B, Lucas S, Warren E, Chaubal M, Kennedy-Hendricks A. Leveraging the affordable housing sector to respond to the opioid crisis. *Public Health Rep*. 2022;137(3):414–419. https://doi.org/10.1177/00333549211007591
10. People's Action. A national Homes Guarantee: briefing book. September 5, 2019. Available at: https://homesguarantee.com/wp-content/uploads/Homes-Guarantee-_-Briefing-Book.pdf. Accessed March 17, 2024.
11. Luo F, Li M, Florence C. State-level economic costs of opioid use disorder and fatal opioid overdose—United States, 2017. *MMWR Morb Mortal Wkly Rep*. 2021;70(15):541–546. https://doi.org/10.15585/mmwr.mm7015a1
12. Macmadu A, Berk J, Kaplowitz E, Mercedes M, Rich JD, Brinkley-Rubinstein L. COVID-19 and mass incarceration: a call for urgent action. *Lancet Public Health*. 2020;5(11):e571–e572. https://doi.org/10.1016/S2468-2667(20)30231-0

Expanding Access to Medications for Opioid Use Disorder: Federal Policy Is Only a Part of the Solution

Omeid Heidari, PhD, MPH, ANP-C, and Caleb J. Banta-Green, PhD, MPH, MSW

ABOUT THE AUTHORS

Omeid Heidari is with the Department of Child, Family, and Population Health Nursing, School of Nursing, University of Washington, Seattle. Caleb J. Banta-Green is with the Department of Psychiatry and Behavioral Sciences, School of Medicine, and the Departments of Health Systems and Population Health, and Epidemiology, School of Public Health, University of Washington, Seattle.

See also Opioids, COVID-19, & Fatal Overdoses, pp. 690–722.

The medications for opioid use disorder, methadone and buprenorphine, are lifesaving and support recovery from opioid use disorder (OUD). Although federal and state policy in the United States has made it difficult for practitioners to prescribe these medications, some recent policy changes have begun to remedy this and make buprenorphine more accessible. In an article in this issue of *AJPH*, Xiong et al. (p. 696) demonstrate this. Their findings show that federal policies to make buprenorphine accessible to people with OUD—in particular, the Comprehensive Addiction and Recovery Act (CARA) and the Substance Use Disorder Prevention That Promotes Opioid Recovery and Treatment for Patients and Communities (SUPPORT) Act—did increase prescribing overall. However, their findings highlight other trends. Although nurse practitioners (NPs) and physician associates (PAs; also called physician assistants) increased their prescribing per month following the passage of CARA and SUPPORT, rates of prescribing among physicians declined.

Although we agree with many of the findings of Xiong et al. and their implications, including that federal policy alone cannot solve issues with buprenorphine access and reaching saturation for this medication, we also believe that other contextual factors help explain why physician rates of prescribing have declined and why more robust policy solutions are needed to address the ongoing overdose crisis. We address implications from several perspectives: clinical, training, implementation supports, care models, and settings.

Firstly, NP and PA prescribers are willing to prescribe buprenorphine for opioid use disorder; given the potentially greater accessibility of these prescribers, this is most welcome. The decline in physician prescribing is concerning because the overall treatment gap between diagnosed and treated OUD remains very large and the scale of morbidity and mortality requires all hands on deck to contribute. As Xiong et al. note, the decrease in physician prescribing can be associated with role shifting. This could be the case in practices where, before the passage of CARA, physicians prescribed buprenorphine for patients whose care was otherwise managed by an NP or PA, who then filled that role after the passage of CARA.[1] However, role shifting likely only explains part of the associated physician decreases in buprenorphine prescribing and points to a larger access problem. For example, one study found that in rural areas, NPs and PAs accounted for over half of the increase in waivered providers.[2] Although there has been improved buprenorphine access since the passage of CARA (NPs and PAs newly prescribing buprenorphine accounted for a 36% decrease in the number of US counties without a single buprenorphine prescriber), and prescribing via telehealth has been associated with increased buprenorphine initiation, there still remains a larger issue of buprenorphine access and retention.

The monthly mean number of patients prescribed buprenorphine increased during the Drug Addiction Treatment Act (DATA), CARA, and SUPPORT time periods of this study (January 2012–February 2020) but stagnated during the COVID period (March 2020–December 2022). If all provider types are prescribing to the same "pool" of patients without significant growth, it can indicate that access barriers still exist. The X waiver is one potential area where we can learn that gatekeeping medications for opioid use disorder (MOUD) continues to have unintended consequences. Unlike countries such as Canada, England, France, or the Netherlands—where MOUD treatment is much more accessible and utilization rates are therefore much higher—the United States has

AJPH July 2024, Vol. 114, No. 7

had a long history of allowing only specialists to prescribe MOUD, or, in the case of methadone, to dispense under stringent rules for patients. Creating this two-tiered system for prescribing and dispensing made methadone and buprenorphine different. Especially in the case of buprenorphine, legislation made a safe medication so difficult to prescribe that the perception was that only specialists should manage it.

We need to make buprenorphine prescribing an expectation, not an exception, in primary and community-based care. It would be unfathomable for us to not avail ourselves of all available drug classes when treating hypertension or diabetes. The same should be said of methadone. As the "liberate methadone" movement continues to grow in the United States, and the Substance Abuse and Mental Health Services Administration (SAMHSA) has codified flexibilities for methadone take-home doses from the COVID-19 pandemic, accessing this medication should be easier.[3] We have the tools and can learn from best practices in other countries. The evidence base is there.

With the removal of the X waiver, clinicians seeking to obtain or renew a Drug Enforcement Administration license are required to complete eight hours of training in the treatment of opioid or other substance use. New clinicians can often fulfill this requirement with content during their clinical coursework and training. Multiple studies have shown that setting substance use disorder competencies in clinical education, which are outlined by SAMHSA, has a positive impact on a clinical student's knowledge and attitudes toward treatment of substance use disorders.[4,5] In particular, interprofessional education with case studies and simulations, and dedicated training in motivational interviewing, are important experiences for clinical education.[6] Care navigators, peers, and nurse care managers as part of a robust clinical support team are invaluable for supporting clients and prescribers.

Although Xiong et al. allude to the potential impacts of nonpharmaceutical fentanyl (NPF) on buprenorphine prescribing, these impacts cannot be understated. NPF arrived in the western United States several years after it hit the East Coast, with substantial increases in mortality roughly coinciding with the onset of COVID-19.[7] This perfect storm had devastating impacts on public health, in part because of the physical, emotional, and financial turmoil resulting from COVID-19 intersecting with the increased challenges of starting on buprenorphine, related to NPF replacing heroin as the primary illicit opioid.[8] Opioid-involved poisoning deaths in Washington State increased from 11.3 per 100 000 in 2019 to 26.3 per 100 000 in 2022; 90% of the deaths in 2022 involved an NPF.[9]

Recent survey and interview data from Washington State indicate that most people who use opioids want to stop or reduce their opioid use, want to utilize buprenorphine or methadone, and often are unable or unwilling to access health care in traditional settings.[10] A new care model provides access to medications at community-based programs, including harm reduction programs providing safer use supplies, and has demonstrated substantial demand, strong engagement, and positive outcomes.[11] This third model, outside of primary care and opioid treatment programs, is needed to help address this massive MOUD treatment and harm reduction gap.

Although prescription monitoring program data are extremely valuable, they also provide very limited information about clients and prescribers, and no information about the care settings or care models. Care settings and models are essential for tracking and evaluating to make buprenorphine available to all who need it. Data systems that integrate health care, first responder, MOUD utilization, and other services data should be strengthened and regularly analyzed, with results widely disseminated.[12]

In summary, federal policy can open doors to broader access to buprenorphine, but specific system and prescriber actions need to happen to take advantage of these new possibilities. Given that MOUD is the most impactful way to reduce mortality, we must make it easier to get than NPF. This means not just increasing access points and providing additional models of care delivery, but a mind shift that MOUD is both treatment and harm reduction. A public health and harm reduction framework would prioritize retaining people on medication as long as they are benefiting from it. The only reason a person should not be on MOUD is because they have been offered it in an accessible manner and made a truly informed decision not to use it. Our best readily available tool to address opioid mortality is MOUD. To shake up our moribund care system and provide people with the medications they need and want, we need prescribers to prescribe and public health to do the necessary education of the public and policymakers—right now. AJPH

CORRESPONDENCE

Correspondence should be sent to Omeid Heidari, PhD, MPH, ANP-C, Health Sciences Bldg, 1956 NE Pacific St, Seattle, WA 98195 (e-mail: oheidar1@uw.edu). Reprints can be ordered at https://www.ajph.org by clicking the "Reprints" link.

PUBLICATION INFORMATION

Full Citation: Heidari O, Banta-Green CJ. Expanding access to medications for opioid use disorder: federal policy is only a part of the solution. *Am J Public Health*. 2024;114(7):693–695.

Acceptance Date: April 23, 2024.

DOI: https://doi.org/10.2105/AJPH.2024.307715

CONTRIBUTORS

O. Heidari and C. J. Banta-Green conceptualized and jointly authored the editorial.

CONFLICTS OF INTEREST

The authors report no conflicts of interest.

REFERENCES

1. Spetz J, Toretsky C, Chapman S, Phoenix B, Tierney M. Nurse practitioner and physician assistant waivers to prescribe buprenorphine and state scope of practice restrictions. *JAMA*. 2019;321(14):1407–1408. https://doi.org/10.1001/jama.2019.0834
2. Barnett ML, Lee D, Frank RG. In rural areas, buprenorphine waiver adoption since 2017 driven by nurse practitioners and physician assistants. *Health Aff (Millwood)*. 2019;38(12):2048–2056. https://doi.org/10.1377/hlthaff.2019.00859
3. Substance Abuse and Mental Health Services Administration. Medications for the treatment of opioid use disorder. 2024. Available at: https://www.federalregister.gov/documents/2024/02/02/2024-01693/medications-for-the-treatment-of-opioid-use-disorder. Accessed March 14, 2024.
4. Muzyk A, Smothers ZPW, Akrobetu D, et al. Substance use disorder education in medical schools: a scoping review. *Acad Med*. 2019;94(11):1825–1834. https://doi.org/10.1097/ACM.0000000000002883
5. Substance Abuse and Mental Health Services Administration. Recommendations for curricular elements in substance use disorders training. 2023. Available at: https://www.samhsa.gov/medications-substance-use-disorders/provider-support-services/recommendations-curricular-elements-substance-use-disorders-training. Accessed March 20, 2024.
6. Muzyk A, Smothers ZPW, Andolsek KM, et al. Interprofessional substance use disorder education in health professions education programs: a scoping review. *Acad Med*. 2020;95(3):470–480. https://doi.org/10.1097/ACM.0000000000003053
7. O'Donnell J, Tanz LJ, Gladden RM, Davis NL, Bitting J. Trends in and characteristics of drug overdose deaths involving illicitly manufactured fentanyls—United States, 2019–2020. *MMWR Morb Mortal Wkly Rep*. 2021;70(50):1740–1746. https://doi.org/10.15585/mmwr.mm7050e3
8. Mariani JJ, Mahony AL, Podell SC, et al. Open-label trial of a single-day induction onto buprenorphine extended-release injection for users of heroin and fentanyl. *Am J Addict*. 2021;30(5):470–476. https://doi.org/10.1111/ajad.13193
9. Addictions, Drug, & Alcohol Institute, University of Washington. Opioid trends across Washington State. Available at: https://adai.uw.edu/wadata/deaths.htm. Accessed March 14, 2024.
10. McMahan VM, Kingston S, Newman A, Stekler JD, Glick SN, Banta-Green CJ. Interest in reducing methamphetamine and opioid use among syringe services program participants in Washington State. *Drug Alcohol Depend*. 2020;216:108243. https://doi.org/10.1016/j.drugalcdep.2020.108243
11. Hood JE, Banta-Green CJ, Duchin JS, et al. Engaging an unstably housed population with low-barrier buprenorphine treatment at a syringe services program: lessons learned from Seattle, Washington. *Subst Abus*. 2020;41(3):356–364. https://doi.org/10.1080/08897077.2019.1635557
12. King County Dept of Community and Human Services. Integrating data to better understand fatal overdoses and service system engagement. 2022. Available at: https://kingcounty.gov/~/media/depts/community-human-services/department/documents/FINAL_integrated_overdose_brief.ashx?la=en. Accessed March 15, 2024.

Federal Impacts on Buprenorphine Prescribing in Washington State, 2012 to 2022

Fan Xiong, MPH, Jillian Jetson, MPH, Cheolwoo Park, PhD, and Chris Delcher, PhD

See also Opioids, COVID-19, & Fatal Overdoses, pp. 690–722.

Objectives. To evaluate changes in monthly buprenorphine dispensation associated with federal prescribing policies in Washington State from 2012 to 2022.

Methods. We conducted an interrupted time series analysis comparing monthly buprenorphine prescriptions dispensed per 1000 population after the Comprehensive Addiction and Recovery Act (CARA), Substance Use-Disorder Prevention That Promotes Opioid Recovery and Treatment for Patients and Communities Act (SUPPORT), and new prescribing rules during the COVID-19 pandemic. Buprenorphine formulated for opioid use disorder was included from the Washington State Prescription Monitoring Program. A log-linear autoregressive model measured linear trend changes.

Results. Physician prescribing increased by 1.63% (95% confidence interval [CI] = 1.41%, 1.85%) per month after CARA with sustained declines after SUPPORT. Nurse practitioner (NP) prescribing increased by 19.48% (95% CI = 18.8%, 20.16%) per month after CARA with physician assistants (PAs) showing similar trends. Following the implementation of SUPPORT, NP and PA trends continued to increase at a reduced growth rate of 3.96% (95% CI = 2.01%, 5.94%) and 1.87% (95% CI = 0.56%, 3.19%), respectively. No prescribers experienced increases during the COVID-19 pandemic.

Conclusions. CARA nearly tripled the buprenorphine prescribing rate. The SUPPORT Act initiated sustained declines for physician prescribing, and the COVID-19 period reversed gains for PAs and NPs. The current opioid crisis requires expanded efforts in Washington State. (*Am J Public Health*. 2024;114(7):696–704. https://doi.org/10.2105/AJPH.2024.307649)

AJPH July 2024, Vol. 114, No. 7

Since 1999, more than 932 000 people have died from a drug overdose in the United States, including 564 000 deaths from any opioids.[1] National provisional data indicate that between April 2021 and April 2022, there was a 6.9% increase in opioid-involved drug overdose deaths, from 76 383 to 81 692.[1] In Washington State, predicted drug overdoses increased by 24.1% from January 2022 to January 2023, the highest percentage increase in the United States.[2] In 2021, the prevalence of past-year opioid use disorder (OUD) in the state was modeled at approximately 2% for residents aged older than 12 years, likely an underestimate.[3–5] In 2017, the estimated cost of OUD in Washington State was approximately $15 billion, ranking ninth among 38 states examined.[6]

Buprenorphine has been an evidence- and office-based medication for treating OUD (MOUD) for at least 20 years in the United States.[7] However, provider uptake has been suboptimal and access to buprenorphine MOUD limited because of mandated patient capacity limits, education requirements, and restricted prescribing waivers to certain qualifying health care practitioners.[8,9] For example, from 2013 to 2016, a study of primary care patients comprising one of Washington State's largest integrated health care providers found only 1 in 5 patients with OUD had documented evidence of MOUD treatment with buprenorphine.[10] Several federal policies were enacted to address these limitations and increase buprenorphine MOUD accessibility.[7]

The first was the Comprehensive Addiction and Recovery Act of 2016 (CARA; July 2016), which allowed waivered providers, previously able to treat only up to 100 patients, to now treat up to 275 patients after 1 year of obtaining a waiver. In addition to this provision, CARA expanded eligibility to nurse practitioners (NPs) and physician assistants (PAs) for prescribing buprenorphine MOUD.[11] The second was the Substance Use-Disorder Prevention That Promotes Opioid Recovery and Treatment of Patients and Communities Act of 2018 (SUPPORT; October 2018).[12] This multifaceted law made it easier to reach treatment capacity, effectively allowing practitioners an immediate 100-patient limit with conditions.[12] In addition to easing Drug Addiction and Treatment Act of 2000 (DATA) application waivers for physicians, the law added clinical nurse specialists, certified registered nurse anesthetists, and certified nurse midwives as additional qualifying health care practitioners (until October 2023). In the years following the passage of CARA, buprenorphine dispensing changed rapidly with nearly all of Washington State's counties experiencing an increase.[13] One report found a 1133% increase in Medicaid beneficiaries receiving buprenorphine in 2018 compared with 2013.[14]

During the COVID-19 pandemic, at least 2 significant changes occurred. The first was the Drug Enforcement Administration's (DEA's) permission for health care providers to prescribe buprenorphine MOUD through telemedicine in March 2020.[15] The second change, in response to an unprecedented number of drug overdose deaths during the pandemic, was removing training and educational requirements from obtaining a waiver.[16]

Although these federal policies all aimed at increasing buprenorphine MOUD access, to our knowledge, no study to date has longitudinally evaluated buprenorphine dispensing over a period covering all of these policies.

We examined trends in monthly buprenorphine dispensing by medical license type and evaluated dispensing changes associated with these key buprenorphine MOUD federal policies in Washington State from January 2012 to December 2022 (11 years).

METHODS

The Washington State Prescription Monitoring Program (PMP) began collecting data on Schedule II to V controlled substance prescription drug dispensed for more than a 1-day supply starting on October 7, 2011. For every PMP dispensing record, required information submitted includes National Drug Codes, dispensation date, written date, days' supply, quantity dispensed, patient residential address, and prescribers' and dispensers' DEA license number.

From the PMP, we extracted all buprenorphine labeled for MOUD records from January 2012 to December 2022 (n = 3 802 464 dispensations); most of these dispensations had 30 or fewer days' supply (99.8%). Because the PMP does not contain diagnostic information, these prescriptions were identified using National Drug Codes (Table A, available as a supplement to the online version of this article at https://ajph.org) and Generic Product Identifier codes from the Washington State Department of Social and Health Services.[14] We excluded buprenorphine prescriptions formulated for pain (n = 296 886), nonhuman animal records (n = 98 315), non–Washington State residents (n = 73 069), and records of poor quality (e.g., unknown zip code, negative age, missing sex; n = 29 825). Demographic information for patients receiving buprenorphine MOUD from 2012 to 2019 is reported elsewhere.[17] Buprenorphine dispensations from federally assisted substance use and mental health treatment, including opioid treatment programs (OTPs), are not reported to the Washington PMP because of federal and state regulations. The Washington State PMP includes mail-order prescriptions, prescriptions paid out-of-pocket, and prescriptions dispensed from Veterans Affairs, Indian Health Services, and military pharmacies.

If available and provided, the Washington PMP collects the National Plan and Provider Enumeration System National Provider Index (NPI) for registered prescribers. We defined medical license type using the primary health care taxonomy from the NPI registry using the provider grouping level of their health care taxonomy code (e.g., allopathic and osteopathic physicians ["physicians"], PAs, and NPs). Approximately 7% of the medical licenses could not be determined.

Statistical Analysis

We calculated monthly sex- and age-adjusted buprenorphine dispensing rates per 1000 using 2012–2022 population estimates based on the Washington Population Interim Estimates (https://doh.wa.gov/data-and-statistical-reports), which are used by the Washington State Department of Health for population rate calculations. We used the 2000 US Census data and direct-standardization methods for sex (male, female) and age categories (< 10, 10–17, 18–24, 25–34, 35–44, 45–54, 55–64, 65–74, and > 74 years). We aggregated the number of buprenorphine prescribers per month by counting the number of unique prescribers with a patient who filled a buprenorphine prescription within the month. Patient counts were not exclusive by medical license type.

The primary analysis was an interrupted-time-series analysis comparing the monthly (n = 132 months) dispensing rates before and after the implementation of CARA and SUPPORT, and the period from March 2020 (COVID-19 public health emergency). Specifically, the periods were DATA 2000 (January 2012 to July 2016; n = 55 months), CARA (August 2016 to October 2018; n = 27 months), SUPPORT (November 2018 to February 2020; n = 16 months), and COVID-19 (March 2020 to December 2022; n = 34 months). The COVID-19 stay-at-home order period was a 3-month period defined as March 2020 to May 2020 (https://www.nytimes.com/interactive/2020/us/coronavirus-stay-at-home-order.html).

In the primary analysis, a log-linear autoregressive model accounted for autocorrelation, seasonality, and any unstable variance in the time series. Our modeling goal was primarily noise reduction rather than a fully optimized model. Autoregressive parameters are not presented but are available upon request. Log transforming the outcome variable (rate per 1000) allowed us to interpret trends as a percentage change. We ran count models of the untransformed outcome to report absolute dispensing changes (Table B, available as a supplement to the online version of this article at https://ajph.org). We measured change using ramping (linear) policy effects and an immediate effect for the COVID-19 emergency period. We conducted the primary analysis by using PROC AUTOREG in SAS version 9.4 (SAS Institute, Cary, NC).

Sensitivity Analyses

Given the relatively high rate of unassigned medical licenses, we examined potential misclassification bias using scenarios whereby 50% and 100% of the missing license types were reallocated to each prescriber type and reran models. We also fitted autoregressive integrated moving average models because of observable nonlinearity in segments of the time series to test whether policy effects were sensitive to autoregressive models. Finally, we calculated monthly percent change by using Joinpoint regression (version 5.0.2) software from the National Cancer Institute to examine whether natural change points in the time series were consistent with a priori selected policy implementation dates.

RESULTS

Table 1 shows the descriptive summary of buprenorphine dispensations reported to the Washington PMP by policy period and medical license type. The average monthly dispensations increased from 16 379 in the DATA 2000 period to 42 662 in the COVID-19 period (March 2020–December 2022). Similarly, the average monthly number of patients and all prescribers increased from 9138 to 28 479 and from 818 to 2570, respectively, over this period.

The mean monthly number of physicians increased from 14 116 to 17 258 from CARA to SUPPORT before decreasing to 14 378 in the COVID-19 period. The mean number of patients per physician also decreased from 12.4 in the CARA period to 10.0 in the COVID-19 period. Meanwhile, the mean monthly number of PAs and NPs increased from 57 to 213 and 112 to 488, respectively, from CARA to COVID-19. The mean number of patients per prescriber also increased from 6.5 to 20.5 for PAs and 6.7 to 17.5 for NPs.

Before the passage of CARA, physicians accounted for 89.9% of dispensed buprenorphine before decreasing slightly to 86.3% when PAs and NPs accounted for 3.3% and 6.8%, respectively, of the state volume. The physician proportion continued to decrease in the SUPPORT and COVID-19 period to 64.5% and 44.6% while PAs increased to 11.1% and 15.9% and NPs increased to 22.7% and 32.2%, respectively. By the end of the study period in December 2022, NPs and PAs accounted for more than half (55.4%) of all dispensed buprenorphine reported to the Washington PMP.

Autoregressive Models

In the immediate period following the implementation of CARA, the state monthly rate of buprenorphine dispensation was increasing by 2.39% (95% confidence interval [CI] = 2.27%, 2.50%; Table 2) or approximately 693.75 prescriptions per month (Table B). Overall, prescriptions dispensed continued increasing but at a lower monthly rate of 0.91% (95% CI = 0.64%, 1.19%) during the SUPPORT period. During the COVID-19 period, this trend began decreasing at a monthly rate of 0.44% (95% CI = −0.59%%, −0.29%). Figure 1 shows estimated and predicted buprenorphine monthly prescribing trends with 95% CIs in Washington State by medical license type from 2012 to 2022.

Physicians

The physician rate nearly doubled after CARA at 1.63% per month (95% CI = 1.41%, 1.85%) but began a downward trajectory after the SUPPORT and

TABLE 1— Buprenorphine Dispensations, Patients, and Prescribers by Prescriber Medical License Type and During Policy Period: Washington State, January 2012–December 2022

	DATA 2000[b] (Jan 2012–Jul 2016; n = 55 mo)	CARA (Aug 2016–Oct 2018; n = 27 mo)	SUPPORT (Nov 2018–Feb 2020; n = 16 mo)	COVID-19 (Mar 2020–Dec 2022; n = 34 mo)
All prescribers[a]				
Dispensations, cumulative no.	900 864	757 935	693 173	1 450 492
Sex- and age-adjusted rate per 1000 population, monthly average	2.4	3.9	5.8	5.5
Dispensations, monthly mean no.	16 379	28 072	43 323	42 662
Patients, monthly mean no.	9138	15 891	24 367	28 479
Prescribers, monthly mean no.	818	1 386	2 037	2 570
Patients per prescriber, monthly mean	10.7	11.0	11.4	10.7
Physicians (MDs and DOs)				
Dispensations, cumulative no.	809 447	653 949	447 336	647 530
% of total dispensations	89.9	86.3	64.5	44.6
Sex- and age-adjusted rate per 1000 population, monthly average	2.1	3.3	3.7	2.4
Dispensations, monthly mean no.	14 717	24 220	27 959	19 045
Patients, monthly mean no.	8240	14 116	17 258	14 378
Prescribers, monthly mean no.	654	1 090	1 356	1 365
Patients per prescriber, monthly mean	12.2	12.4	12.4	10.0
Physician assistants (PAs)				
Dispensations, cumulative no.	4330	24 931	76 643	230 547
% of total dispensations	0.5	3.3	11.1	15.9
Sex- and age-adjusted rate per 1000 population, monthly average	0.01	0.1	0.6	0.9
Dispensations, monthly mean no.	79	923	4 790	6 781
Patients, monthly mean no.	61	521	2 650	4 463
Prescribers, monthly mean no.	19	57	170	213
Patients per prescriber, monthly mean	2.9	6.5	14.6	20.5
Nurse practitioners (NPs)				
Dispensations, cumulative no.	3 705	51 792	157 107	466 980
% of total dispensations	0.4	6.8	22.7	32.2
Sex- and age-adjusted rate per 1000 population, monthly average	0.01	0.3	1.3	1.8
Dispensations, monthly mean no.	67	1 918	9 819	13 735
Patients, monthly mean no.	50	1 036	5 380	8 752
Prescribers, monthly mean no.	21	112	352	488
Patients per prescriber, monthly mean	2.0	6.7	14.5	17.5

Note. CARA = Comprehensive Recovery and Addiction Act; COVID-19 = coronavirus 2019 public health emergency; DATA 2000 = Drug Addiction and Treatment Act of 2000; SUPPORT = Substance Use-Disorder Prevention That Promotes Opioid Recovery and Treatment of Patients and Communities Act.
Source. Washington Prescription Monitoring Program Data, January 2012–December 2022.
[a]Of buprenorphine prescriptions, 6% were missing medical license type from January 2012 to December 2022.
[b]Washington State has allowed PAs and NPs to prescribe controlled substances since at least 2010. The small numbers of buprenorphine prescriptions attributed to PAs and NPs in the DATA 2000 period may be off-label prescribing of buprenorphine for pain or other purposes.

TABLE 2— Monthly Sex-Age-Adjusted Buprenorphine Dispensation Rate per 1000 Population by Prescriber Medical License Type During Each Policy Period: Washington State, January 2012–December 2022

Models	Estimated % (95% CI)	P
All prescribers		
DATA 2000	0.64 (0.59, 0.69)	<.001
CARA	2.39 (2.27, 2.50)	<.001
SUPPORT	0.91 (0.64, 1.19)	<.001
COVID-19	−0.44 (−0.59, −0.29)	<.001
Physicians (MDs and DOs)		
DATA 2000	0.81 (0.72, 0.91)	<.001
CARA	1.63 (1.41, 1.85)	<.001
SUPPORT	−1.71 (−2.16, −1.25)	<.001
COVID-19	−1.56 (−1.79, −1.34)	<.001
Physician assistants (PAs)[a]		
DATA 2000	−0.66 (−1.05, −0.26)	<.001
CARA	16.00 (15.02, 16.98)	<.001
SUPPORT	3.96 (2.01, 5.94)	.001
COVID-19	0.11 (−0.98, 1.21)	.84
Nurse practitioners (NPs)[a]		
DATA 2000	0.67 (0.40, 0.95)	<.001
CARA	19.48 (18.81, 20.16)	<.001
SUPPORT	1.87 (0.56, 3.19)	.006
COVID-19	0.34 (−0.39, 1.07)	.36

Note. CARA = Comprehensive Recovery and Addiction Act (August 2016–October 2018; n = 27 mo), COVID-19 = coronavirus 2019 public health emergency (March 2020–December 2022; n = 34 mo); DATA 2000 = Drug Addiction and Treatment Act of 2000 (January 2012–July 2016; n = 55 mo); SUPPORT = Substance Use-Disorder Prevention That Promotes Opioid Recovery and Treatment of Patients and Communities Act (November 2018–February 2020; n = 16 mo). An autoregressive model accounted for autocorrelation, seasonality, and unstable variance in the time series.
Source. Washington Prescription Monitoring Program Data, January 2012–December 2022.
[a]Washington State has allowed PAs and NPs to prescribe controlled substances since at least 2010. The small numbers of buprenorphine prescriptions attributed to PAs and NPs in the DATA 2000 period may be off-label prescribing of buprenorphine for pain or other purposes.

into the COVID-19 period (Figure 1) by −1.71% (95% CI = −2.16%, −1.25%) and −1.56% (95% CI = −1.79%, −1.39%), respectively (Table 1). In sensitivity analyses, even when all missing licenses were assigned to physicians, the slope in the COVID-19 period remained significantly negative (-0.69%; 95% CI = −0.91%, −0.47%; Figure A, available as a supplement to the online version of this article at https://ajph.org).

Physician Assistants and Nurse Practitioners

After the implementation of CARA, the monthly buprenorphine dispensation rate increased significantly for PAs by 16.0% (95% CI = 15.02%, 16.98%) and NPs by 19.48% (95% CI = 18.81%, 20.16%; Table 2). Though rates remained positive (Figure 1), the rates slowed considerably during SUPPORT to 3.96% (95% CI = 2.01%, 5.94%) for PAs and 1.87% (95% CI = 0.56%, 3.19%) for NPs. During the COVID-19 period, the monthly dispensation rate for both PAs and NPs did not change significantly from the SUPPORT period with no meaningful change in the trend (Figure 1).

Sensitivity Analyses

The results obtained from the autoregressive model did not meaningfully change using autoregressive integrated moving average models (Figure A). Besides the physician model and detecting a significant change point for both PAs and NPs approximately 9 and 12 months after the passage of CARA (April and August 2017, respectively), the Joinpoint sensitivity analysis found change points that closely matched policy dates for almost all models (Figure B, available as a supplement to the online version of this article at https://ajph.org). The physician model had several misaligned Joinpoints, which may indicate unmeasured effects or spurious findings.

DISCUSSION

In Washington State, CARA was associated with increased buprenorphine dispensing among all licensed prescribers and for NPs and PAs in particular by increasing buprenorphine patient capacity.[18] However, the steadily increasing physician prescribing rates, partly boosted by Medicaid expansion in 2014,[19] reversed trends after SUPPORT, a decline that continued to December 2022. This change likely represents population-level prescribing role transfers from physicians to NPs and PAs,[13,20,21] who were previously allowed to prescribe controlled substances in Washington State,[22] but restricted from providing buprenorphine

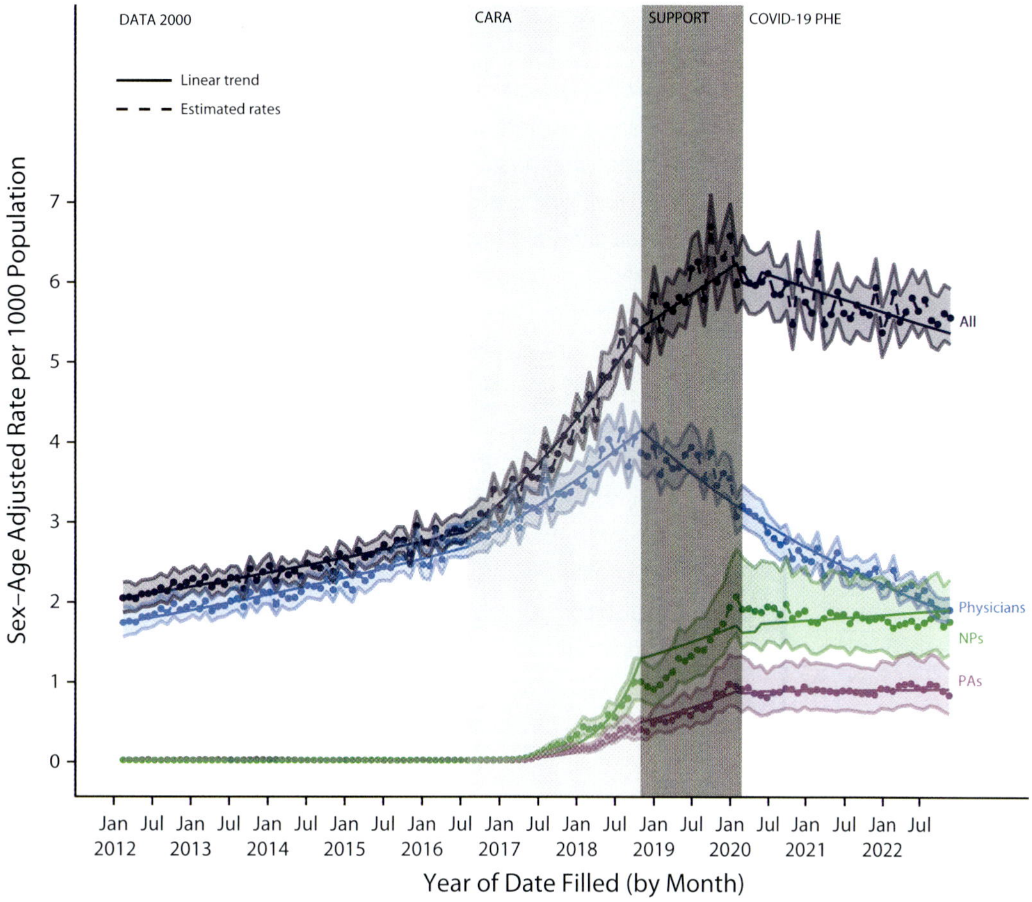

FIGURE 1— **Trends in Monthly Sex- and Age-Adjusted Buprenorphine Dispensation Rate per 1000 Population by Prescriber Medical License Type: Washington State, January 2012–December 2022**

Source. Washington Prescription Monitoring Program Data, January 2012–December 2022.
Note. All = all prescribers; CARA = Comprehensive Recovery and Addiction Act (August 2016–October 2018; n = 27 mo); COVID-19 PHE = coronavirus 2019 public health emergency (March 2020–December 2022; n = 34 mo); DATA 2000 = Drug Addiction and Treatment Act of 2000 (January 2012–July 2016; n = 55 mo); MDs/DOs = physicians; NPs = nurse practitioners; PAs = physician assistants; SUPPORT = Substance Use-Disorder Prevention That Promotes Opioid Recovery and Treatment of Patients and Communities Act (November 2018–February 2020; n = 16 mo). Washington State has allowed PAs and NPs to prescribe controlled substances since at least 2010. The small numbers of buprenorphine prescriptions attributed to PAs and NPs in the DATA 2000 period may be off-label prescribing of buprenorphine for pain or other purposes. Solid lines are autoregressive trends accounting for autocorrelation, seasonality, and unstable variance in the time series of sex- and age-adjusted buprenorphine dispensation rate per 1000 population. Dotted lines are estimated rates from the autoregressive model. Confidence bands shown are 95% confidence intervals of the estimated rates.

MOUD until CARA. The SUPPORT period also marked a slowing of CARA-associated rates for NPs and PAs though prescribing volumes continued to rise. By 2021, the rate of prescribing of NPs and PAs surpassed that of physicians in Washington State, consistent with national research findings that NPs are the highest prescribers by volume[21] and with rapid uptake in neighboring Oregon.[23] The increased uptake by NPs and PAs from federal policy also complements the state's efforts to provide alternative methods to provide MOUD, such as the Washington State Hub and Spoke Model of nursing care.[24] However, our findings indicate that NP and PA expansion is not sufficient to offset the decline in physician prescribing.

The lack of growth in prescribing during the COVID-19 era is concerning but consistent with declines in the national buprenorphine prescribing rates (as of June 2020).[25] Even if we assume that all of the unclassified medical licenses in the PMP are actually physicians, the COVID-19 period rate continued to decrease for physicians. Finally, the lack of sustained growth in Washington State despite several policy attempts to make prescribing easier is consistent with national trends.[26]

The literature on COVID-19–period impacts on buprenorphine prescribing primarily varies according to whether patients are initiating or maintaining prescriptions.[27–30] Some studies found that fewer patients were initiating buprenorphine in an office-based setting and found no decrease in patients in treatment including a telemedicine study using claims from a national sample of commercial and Medicare claims.[27–29,31] Only 1 study from Texas observed an increase in new patients filling buprenorphine prescriptions from 14.3% to 37.6% in the 90 days before and after the national emergency declaration in March 2020, respectively.[30]

The lack of buprenorphine initiation may be associated with the emergence of fentanyl across the United States. For example, the rising number of deaths involving fentanyl have disproportionately impacted non-Hispanic Blacks and Native American/Alaska Native populations.[32] In a recent analysis of national survey data, non-Hispanic Blacks were the least likely to have received MOUD in the past year,[33] and non-White racial populations were less likely to have filled a buprenorphine prescription during the COVID-19 pandemic.[34] Because the Washington PMP does not collect race or ethnicity data, we could not compare our analysis of buprenorphine dispensations in the COVID-19 period to other studies examining racial inequity in receiving MOUD treatment after the emergence of fentanyl.

To our knowledge, this is the first analysis to have measured the sustained impact of these policies on trends in buprenorphine dispensations using PMP data over such an extended period. Thus, we performed a series of consistency checks of our findings against other data sources and states from the published literature. Nationally, prescribing rates per 100 000 increased from approximately 282 in June 2013 to 499 in May 2018.[35] In Washington State, rates were somewhat lower but consistent at 205 and 480 per 100 000, respectively. Our results were consistent with a previous analysis from Oregon's prescription drug monitoring program of NPs, which also did not show any immediate impact but did show a positive increase after CARA.[23] After CARA, Oregon's overall trend increase was 88 prescriptions per month whereas Washington State's was 190.75 prescriptions per month Table B. By the end of 2018, NPs accounted for approximately 18% of all monthly prescriptions in Washington State compared with 14% in Oregon. We also compared the number of PMP patients with an active buprenorphine prescription on March 31 of 2018 and 2019 (16 103 and 19 959) to a previous analysis of retail pharmacy claims data. The counts were reasonably consistent: 14 431 and 16 871 buprenorphine patients, respectively.[5]

Limitations

This analysis used PMP data, which does not include buprenorphine (or methadone) dispensations received by patients in any federally assisted substance use and treatment facilities, such as OTPs. In Washington State, previous research has shown there was approximately 47% more patients receiving any MOUD in an OTP compared with those receiving buprenorphine from retail pharmacies in 2019.[5] In our calculations of OTP data released from the Substance Abuse and Mental Health Services Administration, there was a 115.4% (2021: 10 354) increase in clients receiving buprenorphine on March 31, 2021, compared with March 30, 2019 (2019: 7968)—higher than the 25% (2019: 19 959; 2021: 25 066) increase in PMP patients with an active buprenorphine prescription on those same dates (Table C, available as a supplement to the online version of this article at https://ajph.org). Thus, we cannot account for any increase in buprenorphine dispensations that may have occurred in these facilities.

The findings may not be generalizable to other states because Washington State allows NPs to prescribe without physician oversight, which may have increased prescribing after CARA more rapidly than other states. Our study is not designed to attribute effects to any particular component of these federal policies. SUPPORT had multiple components that could conceivably affect buprenorphine prescribing via multiple pathways, including sending patients to facilities discussed previously. While federal policy changes expanded prescribing authorities, other initiatives, such as those funded by the federal State Opioid Response grants (including the Washington State Hub and Spoke Model), also likely influence access and make it difficult to attribute changes solely to federal policy shifts using Washington PMP data.

Public Health Implications

Buprenorphine is a medication approved for the treatment of OUD, and the decreasing availability in recent periods indicates that removing regulatory barriers, such as waiver capacities and authorizing providers to prescribe, may not sufficiently address the current crisis of opioid-related deaths involving fentanyl starting in the COVID-19 period for Washington State. More research is needed to assess the reasons why buprenorphine prescriptions dispensed may have decreased during the COVID-19 period, especially among physicians, and the impact of health policies that may change MOUD treatment in the near future (e.g., elimination of the X waiver, 28-days take-home supply of methadone from OTPs, and continuing telemedicine flexibility during the COVID-19 pandemic). We emphasize the urgent need for action. The United States has lost more than half a million lives to opioid poisoning since 1999, and each year we see an unprecedented rise in opioid-related deaths. This alarming situation demands our immediate and expanded response to save lives by enhancing access to MOUD, such as buprenorphine and methadone. AJPH

ABOUT THE AUTHORS

Fan Xiong and Jillian Jetson are with the Washington State Department of Health, Tumwater, Washington. Cheolwoo Park is with the Department of Mathematical Sciences, Korea Advanced Institute of Science and Technology, Daejeon, Republic of South Korea. Chris Delcher is with the Institute for Pharmaceutical Outcomes and Policy, College of Pharmacy, University of Kentucky, Lexington.

CORRESPONDENCE

Correspondence should be sent to Fan Xiong, MPH, Washington State Department of Health, 111 Israel Rd SE, Tumwater, WA 98501 (e-mail: fan.xiong@doh.wa.gov). Reprints can be ordered at https://ajph.org by clicking the "Reprints" link.

PUBLICATION INFORMATION

Full Citation: Xiong F, Jetson J, Park C, Delcher C. Federal impacts on buprenorphine prescribing in Washington State, 2012 to 2022. *Am J Public Health*. 2024;114(7):696–704.

Acceptance Date: March 1, 2024.

DOI: https://doi.org/10.2105/AJPH.2024.307649

ORCID iD:
Fan Xiong https://orcid.org/0009-0003-1375-4004

CONTRIBUTORS

F. Xiong acquired the data, conceptualized the study, and initially analyzed the data. C. Delcher contributed further to the study design and analysis as an interrupted-time-series analysis. F. Xiong and C. Delcher wrote the initial draft of the article. F. Xiong, C. Delcher, J. Jetson, and C. Park analyzed the data, interpreted the results, and contributed to the final revision of the article.

ACKNOWLEDGMENTS

This project was supported by grant 2019-PM-BX-0009 awarded by the Bureau of Justice Assistance. The Washington State Department of Health supported this analysis. C. Park's work was supported in part by Basic Science Research Program of the National Research Foundation of Korea funded by the Ministry of Education (NRF-2021R1A2C1092925).

We would like to acknowledge the Washington State Department of Health Prescription Drug Monitoring Program for collecting, cleaning, and providing the data used in this analysis. Additionally, we would like to acknowledge the Washington State Department of Social and Health Services Research and Data Analysis Team for providing the list of National Drug Codes used to identify buprenorphine drugs indicated for opioid use disorder treatment. Finally, we would like to acknowledge the Washington State Health Care Authority State Opioid Treatment Authority for their input on identifying the implementation date of the Comprehensive Addiction and Recovery Act, Substance Use-Disorder Prevention That Promotes Opioid Recovery and Treatment for Patients and Communities Act, and other changes in buprenorphine prescribing policies during the COVID-19 public health emergency period in Washington State. We would also like to acknowledge Eugene Shin for supporting us with creating the data visualization for Figure A (available as a supplement to the online version of this article at https://ajph.org).

Note. The Bureau of Justice Assistance is a component of the Department of Justice's Office of Justice Programs, which also includes the Bureau of Justice Statistics, the National Institute of Justice, the Office of Juvenile Justice and Delinquency Prevention, the Office for Victims of Crime, and the SMART Office. Points of view or opinions in this document are those of the authors and do not necessarily represent the official position or policies of the US Department of Justice.

CONFLICTS OF INTEREST

The authors have no conflicts of interest to disclose.

HUMAN PARTICIPANT PROTECTION

The Washington State institutional review board determined the study exempt from review as a retrospective data analysis for a public health initiative by the Washington State Department of Health.

REFERENCES

1. National Center for Health Statistics. Vital Statistics Rapid Release—Provisional drug overdose surveillance. January 18, 2023. Available at: https://www.cdc.gov/nchs/nvss/vsrr/provisional-drug-overdose.htm. Accessed January 15, 2024.
2. National Center for Health Statistics. Vital Statistics Rapid Release—Provisional drug overdose data. Available at: https://www.cdc.gov/nchs/nvss/vsrr/drug-overdose-data.htm. Accessed August 6, 2018.
3. Substance Abuse and Mental Health Services Administration. Table 27: Opioid use disorder in the past year: among people aged 12 or older; by age group and state, annual average percentages, 2021 and 2022 as measured through the 2021 and 2022 National Survey on Drug Use and Health. Available at: https://www.samhsa.gov/data/sites/default/files/reports/rpt44484/2022-nsduh-sae-tables-percent-CSVs/2022-nsduh-sae-tables-percent.pdf. Accessed June 25, 2023.
4. Thompson K, Barocas JA, Delcher C, et al. The prevalence of opioid use disorder in Kentucky's counties: a two-year multi-sample capture-recapture analysis. *Drug Alcohol Depend*. 2023;242:109710. https://doi.org/10.1016/j.drugalcdep.2022.109710
5. Krawczyk N, Rivera BD, Jent V, Keyes KM, Jones CM, Cerdá M. Has the treatment gap for opioid use disorder narrowed in the US?: a yearly assessment from 2010 to 2019. *Int J Drug Policy*. 2022;110:103786. https://doi.org/10.1016/j.drugpo.2022.103786
6. Luo F, Li M, Florence C. State-level economic costs of opioid use disorder and fatal opioid overdose—United States, 2017. *MMWR Morb Mortal Wkly Rep*. 2021;70(15):541–546. https://doi.org/10.15585/mmwr.mm7015a1
7. Heidbreder C, Fudala PJ, Greenwald MK. History of the discovery, development, and FDA-approval of buprenorphine medications for the treatment of opioid use disorder. *Drug Alcohol Depend Rep*. 2023;6:100133. https://doi.org/10.1016/j.dadr.2023.100133
8. Committee on Medication-Assisted Treatment for Opioid Use Disorder, Board on Health Sciences Policy, Health and Medicine Division, National Academies of Sciences, Engineering, and Medicine. Leshner AI, Mancher M, eds. *Medications for Opioid Use Disorder Save Lives*. Washington, DC: National Academies Press; 2019:25310. https://doi.org/10.17226/25310
9. Saloner B, Karthikeyan S. Changes in substance abuse treatment use among individuals with opioid use disorders in the United States, 2004–2013. *JAMA*. 2015;314(14):1515–1517. https://doi.org/10.1001/jama.2015.10345
10. Lapham G, Boudreau DM, Johnson EA, et al. Prevalence and treatment of opioid use disorders among primary care patients in six health systems. *Drug Alcohol Depend*. 2020;207:107732. https://doi.org/10.1016/j.drugalcdep.2019.107732
11. Substance Abuse and Mental Health Services Administration. Medication assisted treatment for opioid use disorders reporting requirements. Final rule. *Fed Regist*. 2016;81(187):66191–66196.
12. Davis CS. The SUPPORT for Patients and Communities Act—what will it mean for the opioid-overdose crisis? *N Engl J Med*. 2019;380(1):3–5. https://doi.org/10.1056/NEJMp1813961
13. Roehler DR, Guy GP, Jones CM. Buprenorphine prescription dispensing rates and characteristics following federal changes in prescribing policy, 2017–2018: a cross-sectional study. *Drug Alcohol Depend*. 2020;213:108083. https://doi.org/10.1016/j.drugalcdep.2020.108083
14. O'Brien J, Sadwith T, Croze C, Parker S. Review of state strategies to expand medication-assisted treatment: a report to the Laura and John Arnold Foundation. May 2019. Available at: https://www.tacinc.org/wp-content/uploads/2020/02/arnold_state-strategies-to-expand-mat_2019.pdf. Accessed July 26, 2023.

15. Pessar SC, Boustead A, Ge Y, Smart R, Pacula RL. Assessment of state and federal health policies for opioid use disorder treatment during the COVID-19 pandemic and beyond. *JAMA Health Forum*. 2021;2(11):e213833. https://doi.org/10.1001/jamahealthforum.2021.3833
16. Jones CM, Olsen Y, Ali MM, et al. Characteristics and prescribing patterns of clinicians waivered to prescribe buprenorphine for opioid use disorder before and after release of new practice guidelines. *JAMA Health Forum*. 2023;4(7):e231982. https://doi.org/10.1001/jamahealthforum.2023.1982
17. Banta-Green CJ, Hansen RN, Ossiander EM, Wasserman CR, Merrill JO. Buprenorphine utilization among all Washington State residents' based upon prescription monitoring program data—characteristics associated with two measures of retention and patterns of care over time. *J Subst Abuse Treat*. 2021;127:108446. https://doi.org/10.1016/j.jsat.2021.108446
18. Ghertner R. US trends in the supply of providers with a waiver to prescribe buprenorphine for opioid use disorder in 2016 and 2018. *Drug Alcohol Depend*. 2019;204:107527. https://doi.org/10.1016/j.drugalcdep.2019.06.029
19. Saloner B, Levin J, Chang HY, Jones C, Alexander GC. Changes in buprenorphine-naloxone and opioid pain reliever prescriptions after the Affordable Care Act Medicaid Expansion. *JAMA Netw Open*. 2018;1(4):e181588. https://doi.org/10.1001/jamanetworkopen.2018.1588
20. Barnett ML, Lee D, Frank RG. In rural areas, buprenorphine waiver adoption since 2017 driven by nurse practitioners and physician assistants. *Health Aff (Millwood)*. 2019;38(12):2048–2056. https://doi.org/10.1377/hlthaff.2019.00859
21. Larochelle MR, Jones CM, Zhang K. Change in opioid and buprenorphine prescribers and prescriptions by specialty, 2016–2021. *Drug Alcohol Depend*. 2023;248:109933. https://doi.org/10.1016/j.drugalcdep.2023.109933
22. Gadbois EA, Miller EA, Tyler D, Intrator O. Trends in state regulation of nurse practitioners and physician assistants, 2001 to 2010. *Med Care Res Rev*. 2015;72(2):200–219. https://doi.org/10.1177/1077558714563763
23. Klein TA, Geddes J, Hartung D. The geographic impact of buprenorphine expansion to nurse practitioner prescribers in Oregon. *J Rural Health*. 2022;38(1):112–119. https://doi.org/10.1111/jrh.12538
24. Reif S, Brolin MF, Stewart MT, Fuchs TJ, Speaker E, Mazel SB. The Washington State Hub and Spoke Model to increase access to medication treatment for opioid use disorders. *J Subst Abuse Treat*. 2020;108:33–39. https://doi.org/10.1016/j.jsat.2019.07.007
25. Nguyen TD, Gupta S, Ziedan E, et al. Assessment of filled buprenorphine prescriptions for opioid use disorder during the coronavirus disease 2019 pandemic. *JAMA Intern Med*. 2021;181(4):562–565. https://doi.org/10.1001/jamainternmed.2020.7497
26. Stringfellow EJ, Lim TY, Dong H, Zhang Z, Jalali MS. The association between longitudinal trends in receipt of buprenorphine for opioid use disorder and buprenorphine-waivered providers in the United States. *Addiction*. 2023;118(11):2215–2219. https://doi.org/10.1111/add.16291
27. Huskamp HA, Busch AB, Uscher-Pines L, Barnett ML, Riedel L, Mehrotra A. Treatment of opioid use disorder among commercially insured patients in the context of the COVID-19 pandemic. *JAMA*. 2020;324(23):2440–2442. https://doi.org/10.1001/jama.2020.21512
28. Chua KP, Nguyen TD, Zhang J, Conti RM, Lagisetty P, Bohnert AS. Trends in buprenorphine initiation and retention in the United States, 2016–2022. *JAMA*. 2023;329(16):1402–1404. https://doi.org/10.1001/jama.2023.1207
29. Currie JM, Schnell MK, Schwandt H, Zhang J. Prescribing of opioid analgesics and buprenorphine for opioid use disorder during the COVID-19 pandemic. *JAMA Netw Open*. 2021;4(4):e216147. https://doi.org/10.1001/jamanetworkopen.2021.6147
30. Cance JD, Doyle E. Changes in outpatient buprenorphine dispensing during the COVID-19 pandemic. *JAMA*. 2020;324(23):2442–2444. https://doi.org/10.1001/jama.2020.22154
31. Hailu R, Mehrotra A, Huskamp HA, Busch AB, Barnett ML. Telemedicine use and quality of opioid use disorder treatment in the US during the COVID-19 pandemic. *JAMA Netw Open*. 2023;6(1):e2252381. https://doi.org/10.1001/jamanetworkopen.2022.52381
32. Spencer M, Warner M, Cisewski J, et al. Estimates of drug overdose deaths involving fentanyl, methamphetamine, cocaine, heroin, and oxycodone: United States, 2021. Hyattsville, MD: National Center for Health Statistics; 2023. https://doi.org/10.15620/cdc:125504
33. Jones CM, Han B, Baldwin GT, Einstein EB, Compton WM. Use of medication for opioid use disorder among adults with past-year opioid use disorder in the US, 2021. *JAMA Netw Open*. 2023;6(8):e2327488. https://doi.org/10.1001/jamanetworkopen.2023.27488
34. Nguyen T, Ziedan E, Simon K, et al. Racial and ethnic disparities in buprenorphine and extended-release naltrexone filled prescriptions during the COVID-19 pandemic. *JAMA Netw Open*. 2022;5(6):e2214765. https://doi.org/10.1001/jamanetworkopen.2022.14765
35. Knudsen HK, Hartman J, Walsh SL. The effect of Medicaid expansion on state-level utilization of buprenorphine for opioid use disorder in the United States. *Drug Alcohol Depend*. 2022;232:109336. https://doi.org/10.1016/j.drugalcdep.2022.109336

Spatial Heterogeneity in Fatal Overdose Rate Trends in Mexican Cities: 2005–2021

Rosie Mae Henson, PhD, MPH, Pricila H. Mullachery, PhD, MPH, Andrés Sánchez-Pájaro, MD, MSc, Copytzy Cruz-Cruz, PhD, Usama Bilal, MD, PhD, MPH, Brent Langellier, PhD, MA, and Tonatiuh Barrientos-Gutiérrez, PhD, MD

See also Opioids, COVID-19, & Fatal Overdoses, pp. 690–722.

Objectives. To describe national and city-level fatal drug overdose trends between 2005 and 2021 in Mexico.

Methods. We calculated fatal overdose rates at the city level in 3-year periods from 2005 to 2021 and annually at the national level for people aged 15 to 64 years in Mexico. We calculated rate differences and rate ratios for each city between periods.

Results. The national fatal overdose rate was 0.53 overdose deaths per 100 000 population and was almost twice as high in urban than in nonurban areas. The national fatal overdose rate was stable over the period 2005 to 2014 and increased monotonically to a peak in 2021. Fatal overdose rates varied across cities. Cities with the 8 highest fatal overdose rates in the period were all in states along the US–Mexico border.

Conclusions. Fatal overdoses have doubled over the past 15 years in Mexico. Overdose rates are particularly high and increasing in cities close to the US–Mexico border.

Public Health Implications. There is a need for enhanced overdose surveillance data and coordinated harm reduction strategies, particularly in the northern border region of Mexico. (*Am J Public Health*. 2024;114(7):705–713. https://doi.org/10.2105/AJPH.2024.307650)

AJPH July 2024, Vol. 114, No. 7

National estimates of drug use and harms in Mexico are limited, but available data indicate increases in use, decreases in age at initiation, and increases in prescription and illicit opioid availability. The National Survey on the Consumption of Drugs, most recently administered in 2016, reports that national drug use rates doubled between 2002 and 2016: past year use increased from 1.3% to 2.9% and lifetime use from 5% to 10.3%.[1] The median age of drug use initiation has been trending younger in Mexico: from 20.6 years in 2002 to 17.8 years in 2016.[1] Compared with national rates of drug use and related harms, those in the US–Mexico border region, particularly northwest Mexico, have long been significantly higher.[2]

Fatal drug overdose encompasses mortality from the misuse of any type of drug, typically psychoactive substances,[3] and often from a lack of overdose reversal intervention.[4] Fatal drug overdose rates have increased in several countries over recent decades,[5] but trends have not been described for most countries, including Mexico. A 2022 report, using 2016 survey data from people who inject drugs aged 15 to 64 years, estimated the national fatal drug overdose rate in Mexico as between 0.20 and 1.54 deaths per 100 000 population.[6]

Historically, Mexico has been a country of low-level opioid use. However, multiple factors have emerged and converged since 2015, increasing opioid use and overdose risk.[7] These factors are concentrated in the northern border region and include greater availability of psychoactive drugs from US-bound cocaine and synthetic opioid trafficking, regional methamphetamine production and cross-border pharmaceutical opioid access,[8–10] high levels of policing,[11] and strong social and economic ties to the United States during its opioid epidemic.[12,13]

The severity of drug use harms has escalated in recent years, owing in part to the increased presence of, and unknowing exposure to, fentanyl in the local drug supply.[11,14–17] In 2019, fentanyl checking found that 93% of white powder heroin samples in Tijuana contained fentanyl,[14] and a harm reduction program in Mexicali observed a 30% increase in overdoses between 2019 and 2021.[17] Fentanyl seizures also increased significantly in this period. In 2016, Mexican officials seized 15 kilograms (kg) of fentanyl.[18] Between 2017 and 2019 growth was significant, and in the period 2020 to 2022, fentanyl seizures increased exponentially to 1851 kg.[18] In 2023, more fentanyl was seized in 1 operation than in the entire period 2016 to 2019.[18]

Implementation of a national harm reduction strategy in Mexico is still pending.[19,20] In 2020, the federal government issued guidance on the integration of harm reduction into systems of care,[21] but a legal framework for harm reduction did not emerge until reform of the General Law on Mental Health in 2022.[22] This reform made explicit that harm reduction must be integrated into the provision of services for people who use drugs.[22] In 2023, the National Commission for Mental Health and Addictions (Comisión Nacional de Salud Mental y Adicciones [CONASAMA]; https://bit.ly/3Ju5If5) was created as a result of reconfiguration in the Ministry of Health and empowered to develop a national strategy in the field of mental health and addiction, including the provision of harm reduction services.[23] To date, however, no concrete policy has been operationalized.

The increased public health risks associated with fentanyl require a systematic and evidence-based response to prevent overdose deaths in Mexican cities. Epidemiological data on fatal drug overdose allows us to understand overdose risk factors, including how they are patterned geographically and socially, and is necessary to inform opioid overdose prevention, harm reduction, and treatment strategies in Mexico.

OBJECTIVES

We sought to fill knowledge gaps about fatal drug overdose trends in Mexico, including by providing estimates of fatal overdose rates and trends at the city level using mortality records. This information can aid in the development and implementation of targeted, evidence-based practices that prevent fatal and nonfatal overdose and link high-risk populations to harm reduction and treatment services at multiple ecological levels. Our objective was to describe the geographic and temporal variability in overdose mortality rates in Mexico from 2005 to 2021.

METHODS

We used data (Appendix Table A, available as a supplement to the online version of this article at http://www.ajph.org) compiled and harmonized by the SALURBAL (Salud Urbana en America Latina, or Urban Health in Latin America) project.[24] SALURBAL is a research project with teams across Latin America and the United States that study the effects of urban environments on population health.[25] Specifically, SALURBAL obtained mortality data for all deaths in Mexico from 2005 to 2021 from the Instituto Nacional de Estadística, Geografia e Informatica (INEGI). These data include age at death (in 5-year age groups), sex (male or female), underlying cause of death, and municipality where the decedent lived.

Underlying cause of death is recorded using *International Classification of Diseases, 10th Revision* (*ICD-10*; Geneva, Switzerland: World Health Organization; 1992) codes. We excluded records without decedents' place of residence (0.83% of records during the study period).[26] We obtained population projections and intercensal estimates for Mexico from INEGI and the Consejo Nacional de Población, including population counts by 5-year age groups, sex (male or female), and municipality of residence for individuals aged 0 to 65 years for the period 2005 to 2021.

Fatal Drug Overdose

We defined fatal drug overdose based on *ICD-10* codes for drug-involved causes of death. To determine which set of *ICD-10* codes to include in the definition of fatal overdose, we conducted a search of the literature on drug-involved or overdose mortality and hospitalization to determine best practice (Appendix Table B, available as a supplement to the online version of this article at http://www.ajph.org). *ICD-10* codes for injuries have an underlying cause (X and Y codes, indicating mechanism [e.g., drug or firearms] and intent [e.g., accidental or self-harm]) and a contributing cause (T and S codes, e.g., agent [e.g., opiates or stimulants]). *ICD-10* codes for drug use disorders (F codes) are categorized as "mental and behavioral disorders" but are often also included in measures of drug-involved poisoning or overdose. Additional *ICD-10* codes describing drug-involved outcomes are less commonly included in measures of drug-involved overdose and include an array of what are categorized as "other drug-induced causes or adverse effects" (Appendix Table B provides codes included in this category).

Because of major limitations in the coding of drug-involved deaths in Mexico, including a lack of formal testing for potential illicit drug presence,[27,28] the measure of overdose used in this study includes all drug-involved *ICD-10* codes within the categories of "overdose," "mental and behavioral disorders," and "other drug-induced causes or adverse effects" to account for potential coding of these deaths to a wider range of *ICD-10* codes. We redistributed ill-defined injury codes (X59, X84, Y09, and Y34) to other injury codes proportionally based on age and sex.[29] Still, these data likely underestimated drug-involved deaths in Mexico. Alcohol-related causes of death are described in Appendix Table B to provide a complete description of substance use codes but are excluded from this analysis because of the meaningful difference in rates of alcohol use in Mexico compared with drug use, as well as our focus on addressing a gap in knowledge about drug misuse and overdose trends in Mexico.

Analysis

This study is an ecological analysis. We aggregated death-level microdata for fatal overdoses to the municipality level as counts of fatal drug overdose events per municipality, restricting deaths to those aged 15 to 64 years, as this is the age group most likely to experience a drug-involved poisoning.[3] We linked these data to population count data per municipality, also restricted to those aged 15 to 64 years.

We conducted this analysis at 3 geographical scales: national, urban versus nonurban, and specific cities. First, we aggregated counts of drug-involved deaths and population counts across all municipalities in Mexico to compute national fatal overdose rates. These rates were calculated annually, and we calculated 95% confidence intervals (CIs) using a Poisson SE.

Second, we classified municipalities as urban or nonurban based on whether the municipality was part of the SALURBAL study.[24] Briefly, SALURBAL defined urban areas as aggregations of municipalities that overlap with the urban extent, as observed in 2010 satellite imagery of cities with 100 000 residents or more.[24] We then aggregated yearly counts of drug-involved deaths and population counts by urban versus nonurban status and computed fatal overdose rates and 95% CIs.

Third, we aggregated counts of drug-involved deaths and population counts to the city level and calculated city-level fatal overdose rates and 95% CIs. We computed an overall rate for the 2005 to 2021 period and for six 3-year periods (2-year for the final period): 2005 to 2007, 2008 to 2010, 2011 to 2013, 2014 to 2016, 2017 to 2019, and 2020 to 2021. These periods align with trends observed in changes in US overdose rates over the entire period, helping to smooth year-to-year variability given the rarity of events, particularly at the city level. To measure absolute and relative changes in city-level fatal overdose rates, we computed rate differences and rate ratios (RRs) between 2 sets of periods: between 2005 to 2007 and 2017 to 2019 and between 2017 to 2019 and 2020 to 2021. We chose these periods to separate overall secular trends (2005–2007 to 2017–2019) from changes during the COVID-19 pandemic (2017–2019 to 2020–2021). We used longitudinal mixed models with a random intercept for city and robust SEs to test whether changes in fatal overdose rates between these periods were statistically significant. We conducted the statistical analyses using STATA version 15 (StataCorp, College Station, TX).

RESULTS

The national fatal overdose rate among people aged 15 to 64 years was 0.53 overdose deaths per 100 000 inhabitants over the period 2005 to 2021 (Figure 1). National rates were stable from 2005 to 2014, when a monotonic increase started: from 0.44 to 0.79 fatal overdoses per 100 000 from 2014 to 2021 (a 79% increase over 8 years). There was a much higher rate in urban (0.60 per 100 000) than in nonurban (0.37 per 100 000) areas. Although the recent increases occurred in both urban (84% increase from 2014 to 2021) and nonurban (65% increase) areas, increases over the whole period were steeper in urban areas, as rates were similar during the 2000s and started separating in the early 2010s.

City-Level Fatal Overdose Rates

Fatal overdose rates varied widely across cities over the period 2005 to 2021, ranging from a high of 9.84 overdose deaths per 100 000 population in San Luis Rio Colorado (Sonora) to 0.05 in San Juan Bautista Tuxtepec (Oaxaca; Appendix Table C, available as a supplement to the online version of this article at http://www.ajph.org). Geographically, there is a trend of higher overdose fatality rates in northwestern cities, which decreases progressively moving southeast across the country (Figure 2; Appendix Figure A, available as a supplement to the online version of this article at http://www.ajph.org). Of the 15 cities with the highest overdose rates in

AJPH July 2024, Vol. 114, No. 7

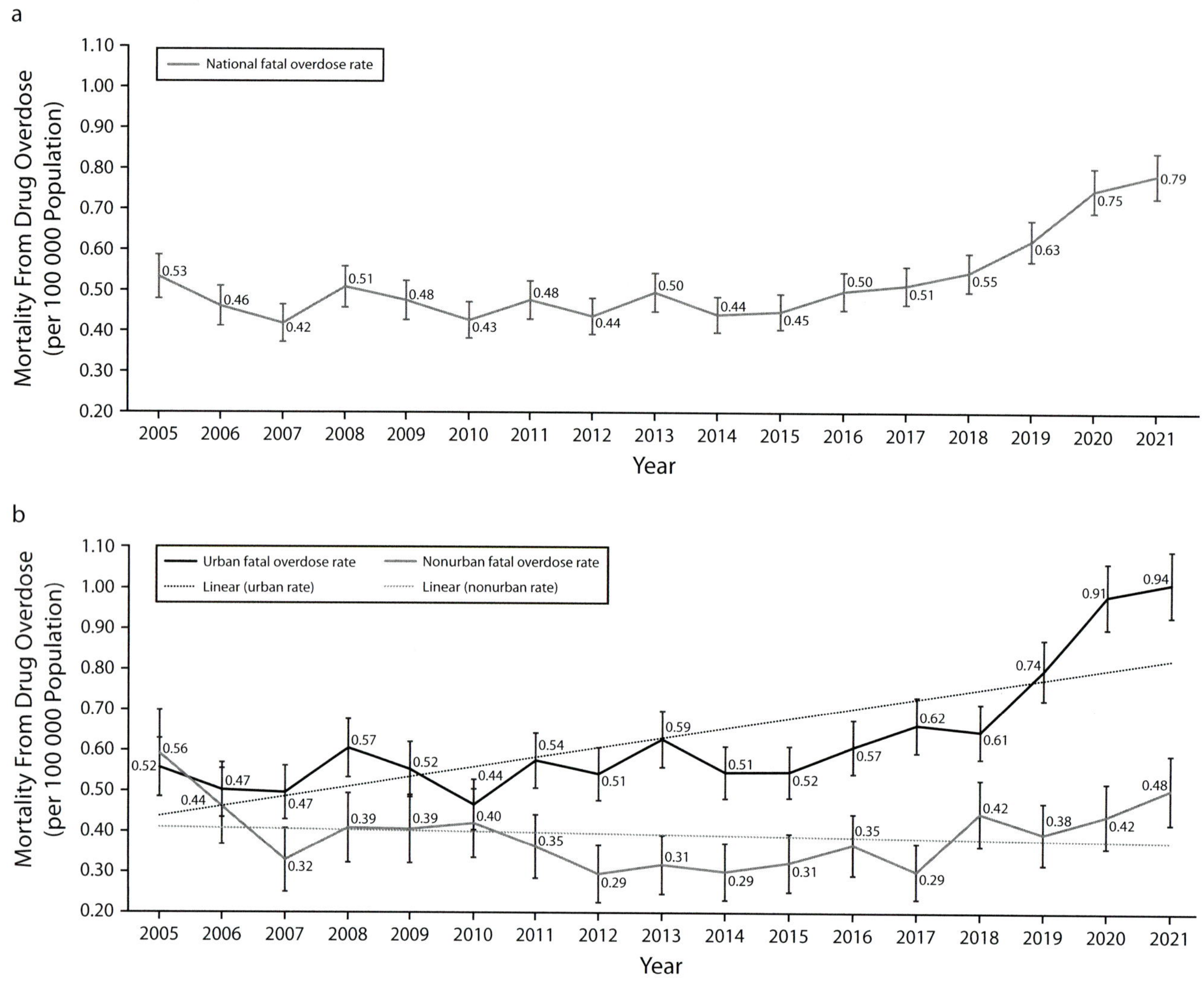

FIGURE 1— Fatal Drug Overdose Rate Trends in Mexico Among People Aged 15–64 Years (a) Nationally and (b) Stratified by Urbanicity: 2005–2021

Note. Whiskers represent 95% confidence intervals. Dotted lines are linear fits representing the slope over the 2005–2021 period.

the period, 11 are in the 4 westernmost states bordering the United States (Sonora, Chihuahua, Baja California, and Coahuila; Table 1) and 5 of these cities are located on the border.

Temporal Trends

We also found wide variation in fatal overdose rates over time (Figure 3; Appendix Figure B, available as a supplement to the online version of this article at http://www.ajph.org). In urban areas, fatal overdose rates increased by 0.17 deaths per 100 000 inhabitants between the first (2005–2007) and the fifth (2017–2019) period of observation and further increased by 0.27 deaths per 100 000 population between the fifth (2017–2019) and the final (2020–2021) period (Appendix Table D, available as a supplement to the online version of this article at http://www.ajph.org).

These changes represented a 35% (RR = 1.35; 95% CI = 1.23, 1.48) and 40% (RR = 1.40; 95% CI = 1.29, 1.52) relative increase from 2005 to 2007 to 2017 to 2019 and from 2017 to 2019 to 2020 to 2021, respectively. These changes followed a similar spatial patterning as overall rates, with larger absolute and relative increases in cities in the northwestern parts of Mexico, especially those bordering the United States (Appendix Table E, available as a supplement to the online version of this article at http://www.ajph.org). Increases in fatal drug overdose rates were significant between the periods 2005 to 2007 and 2017 to 2019 ($P = .02$) and between the periods 2017 to 2019 and 2020 to 2021 ($P = .05$).

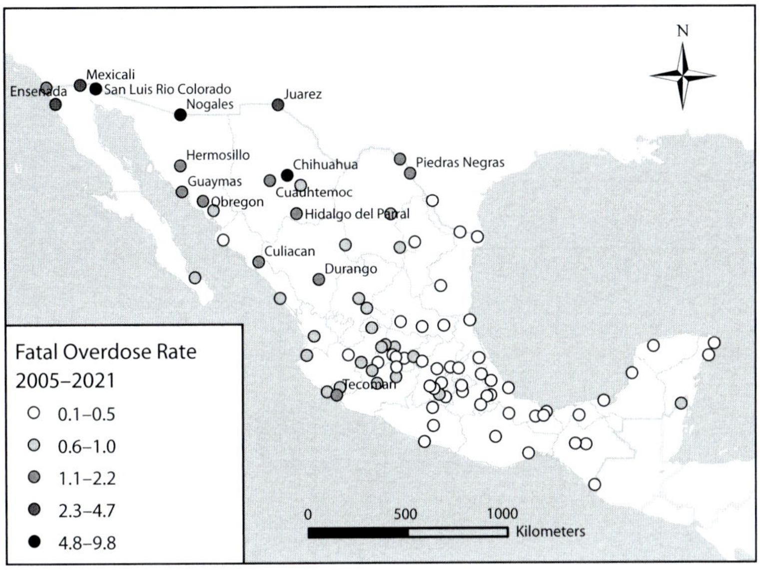

FIGURE 2— Fatal Overdose Rates in Mexican Cities per 100 000 Population: 2005–2021

Note. The sample size was 92 cities. For a full-color version of this map, please see Figure A of the Appendix (available as a supplement to the online version of this article at http://www.ajph.org).

DISCUSSION

In our examination of spatial and temporal heterogeneity of fatal overdose rates in Mexico, we observed 3 key findings. First, national fatal overdose rates in Mexico have increased significantly since 2005, peaking in 2021 so far, with a steep increase from 2014 onward. Second, these increases have been especially steep in urban areas, which had rates similar to those of nonurban areas at the beginning of the study period but almost double by 2021. Third, cities in northwest Mexico had much higher fatal overdose rates and much more steep increases over time.

In Mexico, the national fatal overdose rate was stable over the period 2005 to 2014 and then increased from 0.44 deaths per 100 000 population in 2014 to 0.79 in 2021 (a 79% increase). In the United States, fatal overdose trends remained relatively stable between 2006 and 2013 and then increased from 13.8 deaths per 100 000 in 2013 to 32.4 deaths per 100 000 in 2021 (a 134% increase).[3] Although fatal overdose rates in Mexico are much lower than those in the United States over the same period, the trends are similar.

Urban areas drove increases in national fatal overdose rates, with fatal overdose rate trends in urban areas stable over the period 2005 to 2018 and then increasing to 0.74 in 2019, 0.91 in 2020, and 0.94 in 2021. This represented a 40% increase in fatal overdose rates between the periods 2017 to 2019 and 2020 to 2021 in urban areas. These findings that overdose rates have increased are consistent with findings from an opioid overdose reversal program in Mexicali, which reported a 30% increase in drug overdoses between 2019 and 2021.[17]

Fatal overdose rates were higher in cities in border states and highest in border cities compared with cities in nonborder states. This finding is aligned with historically higher rates of opioid use[2,13] and recently described fentanyl use on the US–Mexico border.[14,15] The observed geographic variation in fatal overdose rates across the country also aligns with the geographic distribution of governmental fentanyl seizures between 2018 and 2023, which occurred in the northwestern states of Baja California (Ensenada, Mexicali, Tecate, Tijuana), Sonora (Opodepe, San Luis Rio Colorado), and Sinaloa (Culiacan, Ahome).[30] These trends suggest that geographic proximity to the United States during its opioid overdose crisis is a risk factor for fatal overdose in Mexico.[7,12,13,18]

Despite these alarming trends, the infrastructure necessary to monitor overdose rates, identify real-time shifts in drug markets, and reduce opioid-related harms in Mexico is insufficient. There is no nationwide overdose surveillance system,[31] and few hospitals and forensic services have the equipment and training necessary to determine drug-related causes of death.[27,28] Evidence-based harm reduction interventions, including community distribution of naloxone, remain criminalized and uncoordinated.[11,17,31] For those seeking treatment, access to evidence-based medications is extremely limited.[31] Our analysis supports local harm reduction practitioners' and epidemiologists' call for a comprehensive, decentralized, and evidence-based policy strategy in response to the emerging overdose crisis along the US–Mexico border.[11,15,17,31]

Limitations

The main limitations of this study are related to the use of vital registration data. Although SALURBAL has imputed missing variables (age, sex) and redistributed ill-defined causes of death,[26,29] there is still the possibility of differential measurement error.

AJPH July 2024, Vol. 114, No. 7

TABLE 1— City-Level Fatal Overdose Rate Trends Over the Period 2005–2021 (Ordered by Highest Fatal Overdose Rate in the Overall Period) in the 15 Mexican Cities With the Highest Fatal Overdose Rates in the Overall Period

		Fatal Overdose Rate per 100 000 Population						
State	**City**	**2005–2021, Overall Period**	**2005–2007, Period 1**	**2008–2010, Period 2**	**2011–2013, Period 3**	**2014–2016, Period 4**	**2017–2019, Period 5**	**2020–2021, Period 6**
Sonora[a]	San Luis Rio Colorado[b]	9.84	4.53	6.28	3.32	7.74	10.97	29.51
Sonora[a]	Nogales[b]	7.55	9.54	4.76	2.76	3.85	9.19	17.59
Chihuahua[a]	Chihuahua	4.74	1.72	3.16	4.30	6.91	4.98	7.38
Baja California[a]	Mexicali[b]	3.46	2.16	1.64	1.97	2.69	4.39	8.69
Baja California[a]	Ensenada	2.90	4.61	2.44	2.78	3.04	3.03	1.35
Chihuahua[a]	Ciudad Juarez[b]	2.24	0.63	3.60	3.37	1.93	1.73	2.11
Chihuahua[a]	Hidalgo del Parral	1.87	1.35	1.27	2.46	0.40	2.69	3.32
Coahuila[a]	Piedras Negras[b]	1.51	0.87	2.17	0.51	0.73	0.92	4.67
Sinaloa	Culiacan	1.46	0.95	1.15	1.86	1.14	2.00	1.59
Colima	Tecoman	1.41	1.92	0.69	2.26	1.22	1.45	0.83
Sonora[a]	Guaymas	1.41	2.51	0.92	0.87	1.66	1.58	0.85
Chihuahua[a]	Cuauhtemoc	1.37	1.39	0.93	0.87	0.84	1.56	2.96
Sonora[a]	Hermosillo	1.23	1.19	0.90	1.06	1.09	1.32	1.95
Sonora[a]	Ciudad Obregon	1.22	0.85	0.67	0.74	1.41	1.24	2.61
Durango	Durango	1.17	0.72	0.82	1.30	1.29	1.22	1.65
All cities (n = 92)		0.60	0.49	0.51	0.55	0.53	0.66	0.92
Nonurban municipalities		0.37	0.43	0.39	0.31	0.32	0.37	0.45

Note. See Appendix Table C (available as a supplement to the online version of this article at http://www.ajph.org) for data on each of the 92 cities.
[a]a state that shares a border with the United States.
[b]a city on the US–Mexico border.

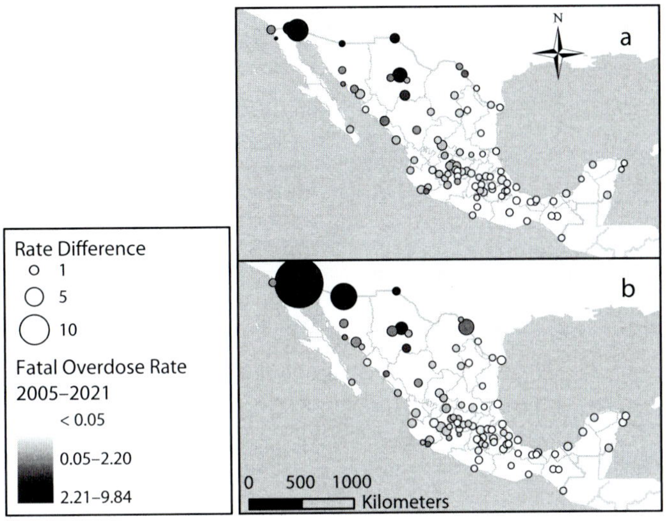

FIGURE 3— Absolute Changes in City Fatal Overdose Rates (a) Before and (b) After Declaration of the COVID-19 Pandemic: Mexico, 2005–2021

Note. Part a shows rate differences between 2005–2007 and 2017–2019. Part b shows rate differences between 2017–2019 and 2020–2021. For a full-color version of this map, please see Figure B of the Appendix (available as a supplement to the online version of this article at http://www.ajph.org).

We corrected for the incomplete coverage of deaths using a city-specific correction factor,[26] but there is the possibility that the coverage of fatal overdose deaths differs from other deaths or that there is miscoding of the cause of death for drug overdose deaths. For example, because drug use is stigmatized, overdoses could occur in isolation and discovery of the decedent could occur after a long time with little indication of cause.[4] In these cases, it is challenging for medical examiners to classify the underlying cause of death as drug involved, particularly without the use of toxicology equipment and the legal and material infrastructure to further investigate the cause of death. This is evident in toxicology data from the Servicio Médico Forense, which in 2021 reported only 1 death from drugs in the states of Baja California, Sonora, Sinaloa, Zacatecas, Nayarit, Colima, Aguascalientes, and Zacatecas but 528 in Chihuahua, 199 in Mexico City, and 283 in Jalisco.[28] This inconsistency in reporting overdose fatalities may explain why the estimated fatal overdose rate for Tijuana, a city known for its high prevalence of drug use, ranked as 16th highest in Mexico between 2005 and 2021.

It is likely that our estimates are a serious underestimation of the true extent of overdose mortality in Mexico. To our knowledge, no data exist to assess whether the extent of undercounts of overdose mortality has changed over time or varies across geographic areas, which would affect our findings regarding secular changes and spatial distribution. This limitation of our study stems from the inadequacy of the current overdose surveillance system in Mexico.

Furthermore, drug-involved events are relatively rare. This limitation does not affect representativeness of the estimates of drug-involved mortality; however, it may affect reliability of the estimates at smaller geographic levels (e.g., municipality). To address this, we pooled 3-year (2-year for the last period) deaths and population. Last, we lacked information on contributing causes (T and S codes), which could have allowed us to explore specific drugs contributing to fatal overdoses, a major and important knowledge gap in Mexico. For example, recent testing for fentanyl in Mexicali found that close to 20% of deaths were fentanyl related.[32]

Public Health Implications

There are several implications of our findings. First, surveillance of drug-related deaths in Mexico is challenging, demonstrating an urgent need for investment in data infrastructure to assess the true magnitude of overdose mortality in Mexico and to monitor trends that indicate a looming overdose crisis. These investments include the use of standardized protocols for coding and reporting drug-related deaths, use of toxicology to identify specific drugs involved in fatal overdose, and the integration of contributory codes on death certificates.[31,33] To account for the gap between overdose events and reporting these events, real-time surveillance systems, including wastewater[34] and street-based[11] drug-checking studies, are necessary for rapid identification of shifts in local drug supply.

Second, the steep increases in fatal overdose we observed emphasize the need for CONASAMA, in partnership with civil society organizations, to coordinate a decentralized, national harm reduction strategy. One of the most effective interventions to prevent opioid overdose deaths is community distribution of harm reduction supplies (e.g., fentanyl test strips, naloxone) paired with education on how to use them for people most likely to witness an overdose.[4,31] In Mexico, however, naloxone is currently classified as a psychotropic drug that requires a prescription and is not available at most pharmacies.[17,31] Our study supports the need for the declassification of naloxone as psychotropic, particularly to address the concerning trend in overdose deaths in the northwest of the country.

Third, future studies should consider the city characteristics that drive fatal overdose rates in Mexican cities. This includes assessing the social, structural, and policy conditions contributing to overdose risk and how these conditions intersect for people in situations of vulnerability,[35] as well as evaluating context-specific interventions to prevent and reverse the occurrence of overdose. This research will be critical for the development of policies and infrastructure to prevent and mitigate overdose risk.

Conclusions

We aimed to understand the temporal and geographic variability in fatal overdose rates in Mexico. We observed an acceleration of fatal overdose rates, particularly in urban areas and in cities closer to the United States. Although the magnitude of the rates in Mexico seems smaller than in the United States, the similarity in temporal trends suggests that important changes in overdose risk are occurring in Mexico, particularly because of the presence and use of synthetic opioids. To prevent an overdose epidemic in Mexico, there is a need for stronger data on drug-related behaviors and harms, harm reduction services prioritizing cities and populations with higher risk, and the expansion of noncompulsory, evidence-based treatment of opioid use disorder. AJPH

ABOUT THE AUTHORS

Rosie Mae Henson and Brent Langellier are with the Department of Health Management and Policy, Dornsife School of Public Health, Drexel University, Philadelphia, PA. Pricila H. Mullachery is with the Department of Health Services Administration and Policy, College of Public Health, Temple University, Philadelphia, PA. Andrés Sánchez-Pájaro and Tonatiuh Barrientos-Gutiérrez are with the Centro de Investigación en Salud Poblacional, Instituto Nacional de Salud Pública, Mexico City, Mexico. Copytzy Cruz-Cruz is with the Servicios de Atención Psiquiátrica, Secretaría de Salud, Mexico City, Mexico. Usama Bilal is with the Urban Health Collaborative, Dornsife School of Public Health.

CORRESPONDENCE

Correspondence should be sent to Rosie Mae Henson, Nesbitt Hall, 3215 Market St, Philadelphia, PA 19104 (e-mail: rhenson@air.org). Reprints can be ordered at http://www.ajph.org by clicking the "Reprints" link.

PUBLICATION INFORMATION

Full Citation: Henson RM, Mullachery PH, Sánchez-Pájaro A, et al. Spatial heterogeneity in fatal overdose rate trends in Mexican cities: 2005–2021. *Am J Public Health*. 2024;114(7):705–713.

Acceptance Date: March 1, 2024.

DOI: https://doi.org/10.2105/AJPH.2024.307650

ORCID iDs:

Rosie Mae Henson https://orcid.org/0000-0002-8099-1080

Brent Langellier https://orcid.org/0000-0002-2136-9486

CONTRIBUTORS

R. M. Henson led study design, data analysis, and writing. R. M. Henson, U. Bilal, and T. Barrientos-Gutiérrez conceptualized the study. P. H. Mullachery and U. Bilal contributed to study design. P. H. Mullachery, U. Bilal, and B. Langellier contributed to data analysis. A. Sánchez-Pájaro, C. Cruz-Cruz, and T. Barrientos-Gutiérrez led interpretation of results and implications. All authors contributed to writing and revising the article.

ACKNOWLEDGMENTS

This project was supported by the Wellcome Trust initiative Our Planet, Our Health (grant 205177/Z/16/Z). R. M. Henson was partially supported by the National Institute on Minority Health and Health Disparities (award T37MD01425). P. H. Mullachery and U. Bilal were also supported by the Office of the Director of the National Institutes of Health (award DP5OD26429).

The authors acknowledge Steven Melly and Goro Yamada for their analytic support as well as the contribution of all Salud Urbana en America Latina (Urban Health in Latin America; SALURBAL) project team members. For more information on SALURBAL and to see a full list of investigators, see https://drexel.edu/lac/salurbal/team. SALURBAL acknowledges the contributions of many different agencies in generating, processing, and facilitating access to data or assisting with other aspects of the project. Please visit https://drexel.edu/lac/data-evidence for a complete list of data sources.

Note. The findings of this study and their interpretation are the responsibility of the authors and do not represent the views or interpretations of the institutions or groups that compiled, collected, or provided the data. The use of data from these institutions does not imply that they have participated in, approved, endorsed, or otherwise supported the development of this publication. They are not liable for any errors, omissions, or other defects or for any actions taken in reliance thereon. The funding agencies had no involvement in the study design; in the data collection, analyses, or interpretation of data; in the writing of this article; or in the decision to submit the article for publication.

CONFLICTS OF INTEREST

The authors report no potential or actual conflicts of interest.

HUMAN PARTICIPANT PROTECTION

This study is exempt from institutional review board review because it involves only de-identified publicly available data.

REFERENCES

1. Encuesta Nacional de Consumo de Drogas [National Survey of Drug Consumption]. *Alcohol y tabaco 2016–2017: reporte de drogas* [Alcohol and Tobacco 2016–2017: Drug Report]. Mexico City, Mexico: Secretaría de Salud; 2017.
2. Borges G, Zemore SE, Orozco R, Cherpitel CJ, Martínez P, Wallisch L. Drug use on both sides of the US–Mexico border. *Salud Publica Mex*. 2018; 60(4):451–456. https://doi.org/10.21149/8603
3. Spencer MR, Miniño AM, Warner M. Drug overdose deaths in the United States, 2001–2021. *NCHS Data Brief*. 2022(457):1–8. https://doi.org/10.15620/cdc:122556
4. Clark AK, Wilder CM, Winstanley EL. A systematic review of community opioid overdose prevention and naloxone distribution programs. *J Addict Med*. 2014;8(3):153–163. https://doi.org/10.1097/ADM.0000000000000034
5. Martins SS, Sampson L, Cerdá M, Galea S. Worldwide prevalence and trends in unintentional drug overdose: a systematic review of the literature. *Am J Public Health*. 2015;105(11):e29–e49. https://doi.org/10.2105/AJPH.2015.302843
6. Magis Rodríguez CL, Villafuerte García A, Angulo Corral MdL, et al. Sobredosis fatales y no fatales por consumo de opioides en el contexto de la pandemia por COVID-19 en el norte de México [Fatal and nonfatal opioid overdoses in the context of the COVID-19 pandemic in northern Mexico]. *Boletín sobre COVID-19 Salud Pública y Epidemiología*. 2022;3(28):7–12.
7. Goodman-Meza D, Medina-Mora ME, Magis-Rodríguez C, Landovitz RJ, Shoptaw S, Werb D.

Where is the opioid use epidemic in Mexico? A cautionary tale for policymakers south of the US–Mexico border. *Am J Public Health*. 2019; 109(1):73–82. https://doi.org/10.2105/AJPH.2018.304767

8. Brouwer KC, Case P, Ramos R, et al. Trends in production, trafficking, and consumption of methamphetamine and cocaine in Mexico. *Subst Use Misuse*. 2006;41(5):707–727. https://doi.org/10.1080/10826080500411478
9. Espino M. Detectan 13 rutas de tráfico de fentanilo, drogamás potente que la heroína [Mexican authorities detect 13 fentanyl trafficking routes]. *El Universal*. January 2024. Available at: https://www.eluniversal.com.mx/nacion/detectan-13-rutas-de-trafico-de-fentanilo. Accessed April 20, 2024.
10. Goodman-Meza D, Friedman J, Kalmin MM, et al. Geographical and socioeconomic disparities in opioid access in Mexico, 2015–19: a retrospective analysis of surveillance data. *Lancet Public Health*. 2021;6(2):e88–e96. https://doi.org/10.1016/S2468-2667(20)30260-7
11. Bailey K, Abramovitz D, Patterson TL, et al. Correlates of recent overdose among people who inject drugs in the San Diego/Tijuana border region. *Drug Alcohol Depend*. 2022;240:109644. https://doi.org/10.1016/j.drugalcdep.2022.109644
12. Borges G, Cherpitel CJ, Orozco R, et al. Substance use and cumulative exposure to American society: findings from both sides of the US–Mexico border region. *Am J Public Health*. 2016;106(1):119–127. https://doi.org/10.2105/AJPH.2015.302871
13. Volkmann T, Shin SS, Garfein RS, et al. Border crossing to inject drugs in Mexico among injection drug users in San Diego, California. *J Immigr Minor Health*. 2012;14(2):281–286. https://doi.org/10.1007/s10903-011-9462-9
14. Fleiz C, Arredondo J, Chavez A, et al. Fentanyl is used in Mexico's northern border: current challenges for drug health policies. *Addiction*. 2020; 115(4):778–781. https://doi.org/10.1111/add.14934
15. Friedman J, Bourgois P, Godvin M, et al. The introduction of fentanyl on the US–Mexico border: an ethnographic account triangulated with drug checking data from Tijuana. *Int J Drug Policy*. 2022;104:103678. https://doi.org/10.1016/j.drugpo.2022
16. Friedman J, Godvin M, Molina C, et al. Fentanyl, heroin, and methamphetamine-based counterfeit pills sold at tourist-oriented pharmacies in Mexico: an ethnographic and drug checking study. *Drug Alcohol Depend*. 2023;249:110819. https://doi.org/10.1016/j.drugalcdep.2023.110819
17. Goodman-Meza D, Slim S, Angulo L, et al. Impact of an overdose reversal program in the context of a safe consumption site in northern Mexico. *Drug Alcohol Depend Rep*. 2021;2:100021. https://doi.org/10.1016/j.dadr.2021.100021 [Erratum in: *Drug Alcohol Depend Rep*. 2022;4:100079].
18. Pérez Ricart CA, Ibarrola García A. La transición hacia el fentanilo: cambios y continuidades del mercado de drogas en México (2015–2022) [The transition to fentanyl: changes and continuities of the drug market in Mexico (2015–2022)]. *Rev Cienc Soc*. 2023;36(53):15–36. https://doi.org/10.26489/rvs.v36i53.1
19. Jargiełło A. Harm reduction model in Mexico's drug policy. *Anuario Latinoamericano—Ciencias Políticas y Relaciones Internacionales*. 2021;11:131–145. https://doi.org/10.17951/al.2021.11.131-145
20. Guerra E, Zwitser G. Civil society organizations and harm reduction policy: the Mexican case. *Contemp Drug Probl*. 2023;51(1):45–64. https://doi.org/10.1177/00914509231214344
21. Secretaría de Salud. Guía breve para la implementación del enfoque de reducción de riesgos y daños con usuarios de drogas [Brief guide for implementing the risk and harm reduction approach with drug users]. June 18, 2020. Available at: https://www.gob.mx/salud/conadic/documentos/guia-breve-para-la-implementacion-del-enfoque-de-reduccion-de-riesgos-y-danos-con-usuarios-de-drogas. Accessed April 20, 2024.
22. Secretaría de Salud. Decreto por el que se reforman, adicionan y derogan diversas disposiciones de la Ley General de Salud, en materia de Salud Mental y Adicciones [Decree by which various provisions of the General Health Law are amended, added, and repealed, concerning mental health and addictions]. May 16, 2022. Available at: https://www.diputados.gob.mx/LeyesBiblio/ref/lgs/LGS_ref131_16may22.pdf. Accessed January 23, 2024.
23. Secretaría de Gobernación. Decreto por el que se crea la Comisión Nacional de Salud Mental y Adicciones como un órgano administrativo desconcentrado de la Secretaría de Salud [Decree creating the National Commission for Mental Health and Addictions as a decentralized administrative body of the Ministry of Health]. May 29, 2023. Available at: https://www.dof.gob.mx/nota_detalle.php?codigo=5690283&fecha=29/05/2023#gsc.tab=0. Accessed January 23, 2024.
24. Quistberg DA, Diez Roux AV, Bilal U, et al. Building a data platform for cross-country urban health studies: the SALURBAL study. *J Urban Health*. 2019;96(2):311–337. https://doi.org/10.1007/s11524-018-00326-0
25. Diez Roux AV, Slesinski SC, Alazraqui M, et al. A novel international partnership for actionable evidence on urban health in Latin America: LAC-Urban Health and SALURBAL. *Glob Chall*. 2018;3(4):1800013. https://doi.org/10.1002/gch2.201800013
26. Bilal U, Hessel P, Perez-Ferrer C, et al. Life expectancy and mortality in 363 cities of Latin America. *Nat Med*. 2021;27(3):463–470. https://doi.org/10.1038/s41591-020-01214-4
27. West BS, Abramovitz DA, Gonzalez-Zuniga P, et al. Drugs, discipline and death: causes and predictors of mortality among people who inject drugs in Tijuana, 2011–2018. *Int J Drug Policy*. 2020;75:102601. https://doi.org/10.1016/j.drugpo.2019.11.009
28. Secretaría de Salud. Sistema de Vigilancia Epidemiológica de las Adicciones: Informe SISVEA 2021 [Addiction Epidemiological Surveillance System: SISVEA Report 2021]. September 2022. Available at: https://www.gob.mx/cms/uploads/attachment/file/760957/informe_sisvea_2021.pdf. Accessed April 20, 2024.
29. Mullachery PH, Rodriguez DA, Miranda JJ, et al. Mortality amenable to healthcare in Latin American cities: a cross-sectional study examining between-country variation in amenable mortality and the role of urban metrics. *Int J Epidemiol*. 2022;51(1):303–313. https://doi.org/10.1093/ije/dyab137
30. Secretaría de la Defensa Nacional. Informe de Labores (2019–2024) [Work report (2019–2024)]. February 1, 2023. Available at: https://www.gob.mx/sedena/acciones-y-programas/informe-de-labores-de-la-sedena. Accessed January 23, 2024.
31. Bejarano Romero R, Arredondo Sánchez-Lira J, Slim Pasaran S, et al. Implementing a decentralized opioid overdose prevention strategy in Mexico, a pending public policy issue. *Lancet Reg Health Am*. 2023;23:100535. https://doi.org/10.1016/j.lana.2023.100535
32. Linthicum K, Blakinger K, Sheets C. Mexico says it doesn't have a fentanyl problem. New data reveal a hidden epidemic. *Los Angeles Times*. July 7, 2023. Available at: https://www.latimes.com/world-nation/story/2023-07-07/mexico-fentanyl-meth-epidemic-data-shows. Accessed January 23, 2024.
33. Davis GG, Cadwallader AB, Fligner CL, et al. Recommendations for the investigation, diagnosis, and certification of deaths related to opioid and other drugs. *Am J Forensic Med Pathol*. 2020; 41(3):152–159. https://doi.org/10.1097/PAF.0000000000000550
34. Cruz-Cruz C, Vidaña-Pérez D, Mondragón Y Kalb M, et al. Medición de drogas ilícitas en aguas residuales: estudio piloto en México [Assessing illicit drugs in wastewater: a pilot study in Mexico]. *Salud Publica Mex*. 2019;61(4):461–469. https://doi.org/10.21149/9819
35. Gonzalez-Nieto P, Salimian A, Arredondo J, et al. Intersections between syndemic conditions and stages along the continuum of overdose risk among women who inject drugs in Mexicali, Mexico. *Harm Reduct J*. 2023;20(1):79. https://doi.org/10.1186/s12954-023-00815-9

State COVID-19 Policies and Drug Overdose Mortality Among Working-Age Adults in the United States, 2020

Douglas A. Wolf, PhD, Shannon M. Monnat, PhD, Emily E. Wiemers, PhD, Yue Sun, MA, Xue Zhang, PhD, Elyse R. Grossman, PhD, and Jennifer Karas Montez, PhD

See also Opioids, COVID-19, & Fatal Overdoses, pp. 690–713.

Objectives. To identify relationships between US states' COVID-19 in-person activity limitation and economic support policies and drug overdose deaths among working-age adults in 2020.

Methods. We used county-level data on 140 435 drug overdoses among adults aged 25 to 64 years during January 2019 to December 2020 from the National Vital Statistics System and data on states' COVID-19 policies from the Oxford COVID-19 Government Response Tracker to assess US trends in overdose deaths by sex in 3138 counties.

Results. Policies limiting in-person activities significantly increased, whereas economic support policies significantly decreased, overdose rates. A 1-unit increase in policies restricting activities predicted a 15% average monthly increase in overdose rates for men (incident rate ratio [IRR] = 1.15; 95% confidence interval [CI] = 1.09, 1.20) and a 14% increase for women (IRR = 1.14; 95% CI = 1.09, 1.20). A 1-unit increase in economic support policies predicted a 3% average monthly decrease for men (IRR = 0.97; 95% CI = 0.95, 1.00) and a 4% decrease for women (IRR = 0.96; 95% CI = 0.93, 0.99). All states' policy combinations are predicted to have increased drug-poisoning mortality.

Conclusions. The economic supports that states enacted were insufficient to fully mitigate the adverse relationship between activity limitations and drug overdoses. (*Am J Public Health*. 2024;114(7):714–722. https://doi.org/10.2105/AJPH.2024.307621)

AJPH July 2024, Vol. 114, No. 7

Drug overdose rates surged in the United States during the first year of the COVID-19 pandemic. Data from the US Centers for Disease Control and Prevention (CDC) show 91 799 drug-poisoning deaths in 2020, up from 70 630 in 2019.[1] However, increases varied geographically, with some states experiencing increases of more than 50% between 2019 and 2020, whereas others experienced small increases or decreases. There have also been large within-state differences in overdose rates.[2] In 2020 these differences continued, with fatal overdose rates for men higher in metropolitan counties and those for women higher in nonmetropolitan counties.[3]

Public health experts raised concerns in the early months of the COVID-19 pandemic about how the pandemic and the policies enacted to stem it might increase overdose risk.[4,5] Several states enacted various policies to reduce the spread of severe acute respiratory syndrome coronavirus 2 (SARS-CoV-2), including policies that limited individual activities (e.g., stay-at-home orders), restricted operations in institutional settings (e.g., substance use treatment services), and closed public transportation and businesses. These restrictions may have reduced overdose risk because of the increasing scarcity and the rising cost of drugs, reduced access to dealers, and increased closures of places where drug use is common (e.g., nightclubs).[6] Alternatively, these restrictions may have increased overdose risk through adverse effects on employment and economic well-being,[7] isolation, and mental health[8,9]; decreased access to treatment and harm reduction services (including difficulty accessing Naloxone)[10–13]; inadequate supply of emergency medical responders[10]; decreased interdiction[14]; and increased solitary drug use, thereby reducing the likelihood of intervention during an overdose.[10]

Working-age adults may have been at particular risk given that they bore the brunt of employment losses, income hardship, and stress from homeschooling and caring for older parents.[11] Given that restrictions on in-person interactions had disproportionate impacts on sectors with high women employment shares and closures of schools and daycare centers increased childcare needs,[15] the relationship between states' COVID-19 policies and drug overdose rates might have varied by sex.

Studies on the effects of stay-at-home orders have generally shown increases in substance use[16] and overdose rates.[17–22] However, studies to date have been limited to specific states or cities or have not used variation in the severity of the mandates or the effects of other policies that were often enacted simultaneously with stay-at-home orders (e.g., school closures). Moreover, to mitigate the adverse effects of the pandemic and associated restrictive policies, many states enacted income support and debt relief policies, such as direct cash payments and eviction moratoria. These policies may have reduced overdose risk by reducing economic stress. Alternatively, the extra income they provided may have increased overdose risk, particularly during a period of severe social isolation, reduced treatment and recovery supports, and a reduction in the quality of the drug supply, all of which may have increased substitution of toxic and adulterated substances.[23]

We assessed the relationship between US states' COVID-19 stringency policies and economic support policies and county-level drug overdose deaths among working-age adults during 2020. These 2 types of policies were most extensively used in 2020, and the year ended with the authorization of the first vaccine approved for widespread use in preventing COVID-19. In addition to considering both policy domains, we advance knowledge by capturing the entire United States and considering a period with substantial variation in the intensity and timing of the policies. Our findings could inform future policy discussions regarding which combinations of policies best prevent overdose risk during a period that requires interventions to reduce infectious disease spread.

METHODS

We obtained 2019 and 2020 mortality files via a restricted data use agreement from the National Center for Health Statistics (NCHS). We identified drug-poisoning deaths using the *International Classification of Disease, 10th Revision* underlying cause of death codes for drug poisoning (X40-X44, X60-X64, X85, Y10-Y14). We computed drug-poisoning death counts by county, month, and sex (men, women) among adults aged 25 to 64 years between January 2019 and December 2020.

Population Counts

We interpolated midmonth county population counts by age and sex from the annual CDC Bridged Race Population Count files[24] and merged them with the death counts. These counts represent the exposure to risk in our regressions.

States' COVID-19 Policies

We used 2 COVID-19 policy indices from the Oxford COVID-19 Government Response Tracker.[25] The stringency index (SI) quantifies the strictness of lockdown policies that primarily restricted individuals' in-person interactions. It incorporates 8 components, such as school and workplace closures and restrictions on gathering. The economic support index (ESI) quantifies income support (e.g., direct cash payments) and debt relief (e.g., eviction moratoria) policies. Table A (available as a supplement to the online version of this article at http://www.ajph.org) provides details of the components and construction of the indices.

Each state has a daily index value between 0 and 100, with higher values indicating broader or more robust coverage. We divided each score by 10 to produce a metric more closely calibrated with patterns of change observed during the period. We calculated monthly averages for both indices, which we merged with the mortality data using a 1-month lag (i.e., we merged policies for March–November 2020 with mortality for April–December 2020).

We addressed associations between state-level COVID-19 policies and county-level drug overdose mortality for several reasons. First, although federal, state, and local governments were all involved in COVID-19–related policies during this period, the rules and procedures for federal policies were uniform throughout the country. Accordingly, we focused on state policies, because states have the primary legal responsibility for enacting pandemic control measures.[26] Although many localities imposed their own COVID-19 policies, there is no national database that provides those policy measures. One study, which compiled the policies of a sample of 171 counties,[27] showed that for numerous specific components of containment, closures, and economic support policies, more than half of the counties studied adopted no measures, effectively ceding policy setting to the state. Moreover, many states preempted local governments from enacting public health emergency policies during the pandemic.[28]

Covariates

We controlled for monthly COVID-19 severity (March–December 2020) in each county's immediate area using the COVID-19 death rate (deaths per 100 000 population) in an area that included all neighboring counties, including counties located in adjacent states. Monthly COVID-19 death counts are from the restricted NCHS files. We also included 2 county-level time-invariant confounders: the percentage of the population in poverty (as revealed in the 2019 American Community Survey) and the percentage of votes received by the Republican candidate in the 2016 presidential election.

We also controlled for county metropolitan status using the US Department of Agriculture Economic Research Service's 2013 Rural–Urban Continuum Codes (RUCC); 2013 is the most recent year for which these codes are available.[29] Metropolitan counties are those assigned RUCCs 1 to 3. Nonmetropolitan counties are those with RUCCs of 4 to 9. We incorporated trends in overdoses specific to every combination of state and metro versus nonmetro category. These area-specific trends served as the baseline from which 2020 deviations were estimated. Together, the county-level covariates and the area-specific trends addressed within-state heterogeneity of drug overdose deaths. Finally, we controlled for calendar months in the multivariable models.

Statistical Analysis

Our drug overdose mortality data covered a 14-month prepandemic period (January 2019–February 2020) followed by a 10-month active pandemic period (March 2020–December 2020), during which all counties were subject to both SI and ESI policy interventions. We used an interrupted time series quasiexperimental design[30] to estimate relationships between outcomes and the SI and ESI policies. This approach assumes that in the absence of COVID-19 and the policy responses to it, pre–COVID-19 trends in overdose mortality would have continued.

The principal threat to internal validity with the interrupted time series design is the possibility that factors other than the intervention influenced the outcome.[30] To guard against this, we implemented a 2-stage multivariable regression approach. In the first stage we used Poisson pseudo–maximum likelihood (PPML) regression[31] to estimate a prepandemic trend for every combination of state and metropolitan status category. The outcome in the PPML model is the count of drug overdose deaths for each county–month combination; the number at risk for an overdose death is reflected by the county population. We used the first-stage model results to compute the expected number of drug overdose deaths in each county for each month beginning with March 2020. These calculations extrapolated prepandemic trends through 2020[32] and served as the counterfactual outcomes for various policy scenarios described later.

In the second stage of the analysis, we used a PPML model of overdose deaths during March to December 2020 as a function of the SI and ESI policies and controls previously described along with the computed number of expected deaths from the first-stage analysis entered as a covariate. Details on the models estimated are available in Appendix A (available as a supplement to the online version of this article at http://www.ajph.org).

We estimated several second-stage models. Model 1 included only SI policies and controls, model 2 included only ESI policies and controls, and model 3 included both SI and ESI policies and controls. We show models 1 and 2 for comparison with our preferred model (model 3), given that some previous studies have not considered both types of policies simultaneously.[33,34] Models 1 to 3 produce a single estimate of each policy's association with drug overdose deaths for the April to December 2020 period. Because the county-level COVID-19 severity variable, included as a covariate in the second-stage estimation, could itself reflect part of the response to the SI and ESI policies, we estimated model 4, which excluded it as a covariate.

We also estimated model 5, in which the association between the SI and ESI policy indices and overdose deaths were allowed to vary by subperiod (April–June, July–August, September–December; Table B, available as a supplement to the online version of this article at http://www.ajph.org). Model 6 is similar to model 3 but combines men and women in a population-level analysis (Table C, available as a supplement to the online version of this article at http://www.ajph.org). We bootstrapped the entire estimation sequence to obtain confidence intervals (CIs) for estimated coefficients using 2000 bootstrap replicates.

Because our outcomes were measured at the county level whereas policies were measured at the state level, there may be some induced correlation of outcomes among adjacent clusters of counties. Our use of area-specific baseline trends, fixed- and time-varying county-level covariates, and bootstrapped CIs reduced inferential problems associated with the spatial clustering of outcomes.

In counterfactual analyses, we computed average values of SI and ESI for the March to November 2020 period to identify states that tended to adopt more versus less expansive values of each policy during the year. We chose states with each possible combination of low versus high levels of SI and ESI to represent the counterfactual scenarios. We used the sequences of SI and ESI policies adopted in 4 specific states to predict overdose deaths using model 3, assuming that all states had adopted each of 4 scenarios: (1) low levels of SI, high levels of ESI; (2) low SI, low ESI; (3) high SI, high ESI; and (4) high SI, low ESI.

RESULTS

We included 140 435 drug-poisoning deaths among adults aged 25 to 64 years (96 856 for men; 43 579 for women), with 75 264 county-months of observations for each sex, covering 2019 and 2020. From March through December 2020, men (women) experienced 47 466 (20 637) drug-poisoning deaths. Figure 1 plots drug-poisoning deaths by month and sex for the United States overall. Similar figures for each state are shown in Figure A (available as a supplement to the online version of this article at http://www.ajph.org). For each sex, the fitted prepandemic trend line is shown (solid lines), with extrapolated points representing the pandemic period (dashed lines). The prepandemic monthly death counts are very close to their respective linear trend lines. The prepandemic upward trend is slightly steeper for men than for women. Finally, a sharp rise in drug-poisoning death rates early in the pandemic is evident and is markedly larger among men than women. Rates for both men and women returned to the extrapolated trend lines near the end of 2020.

COVID-19 policies imposed during March to November 2020 (the period for which they appeared in our model because of the 1-month lag used) ranged from 3.3 (on the 0–10 scale) to 9.3 for SI and from 1.0 to 10 for ESI. The medians during this period were 6.2 and 6.3, respectively; the interquartile ranges were 1.9 and 4.0. Although SI and ESI policy scores for the entire United States rose rapidly beginning in March, SI policies tended to be higher between March and April and again from August onward; ESI policies were higher in May to July. These patterns are shown graphically in Figure B (available as a supplement to the online version of this article at http://www.ajph.org). The corresponding trends for individual states are illustrated in Figure C (available as a supplement to the online version of this article at http://www.ajph.org).

Results from the second-stage regression analysis are shown in Table 1. Model 1 shows that stronger SI policies predicted significantly higher drug-poisoning mortality for men and women, whereas model 2 shows that stronger ESI policies were unrelated to drug deaths. Model 3, which includes both policies, shows that stronger SI policies predicted significantly higher, whereas stronger ESI policies predicted significantly lower, drug-poisoning mortality for men and women. Specifically, a 1-unit increase in SI (corresponding to 10 points on the original 1–100 scale) was associated with a 15% average monthly increase in drug-poisoning mortality for men (incident rate ratio [IRR] = 1.15; 95% CI = 1.09, 1.20) and a 14% monthly average increase for women (IRR = 1.14; 95% CI = 1.09, 1.20). Conversely, a 1-unit increase in the ESI was associated with a 3% average monthly decrease in drug-poisoning mortality for men (IRR = 0.97; 95% CI = 0.95, 1.00) and a 4% decrease for women (IRR = 0.96; 95% CI = 0.93, 0.99). Model 4, which omits the control for county-level COVID-19 severity, does not alter these conclusions.

Model 3 shows that the 2 policies have countervailing relationships with drug-poisoning deaths. This implies that there could be combinations of SI and ESI that offset each other in terms of drug-poisoning mortality. However, no states adopted policy combinations that would have predicted either a decrease or no increase in drug mortality. Indeed, all states enacted combinations of policies that predicted increases, ranging from about 60% to 170%, in drug overdose mortality for men (the relationship was the same for women). These patterns are illustrated in Figure D (available as a supplement to the online version of this article at http://www.ajph.org).

To address the potential for region-specific factors associated with drug overdoses but unrelated to the SI and ESI policies, we conducted 2 sensitivity analyses. First, reflecting historical patterns of the spread of illicitly manufactured fentanyl, we added to model 3 an interaction between time (the month effects) and an indicator of states that lie east of the Mississippi River. Second, we introduced additional underlying trend lines, 1 for each of the 9 RUCC codes (in place of the metro vs nonmetro distinction used in model 3). Neither

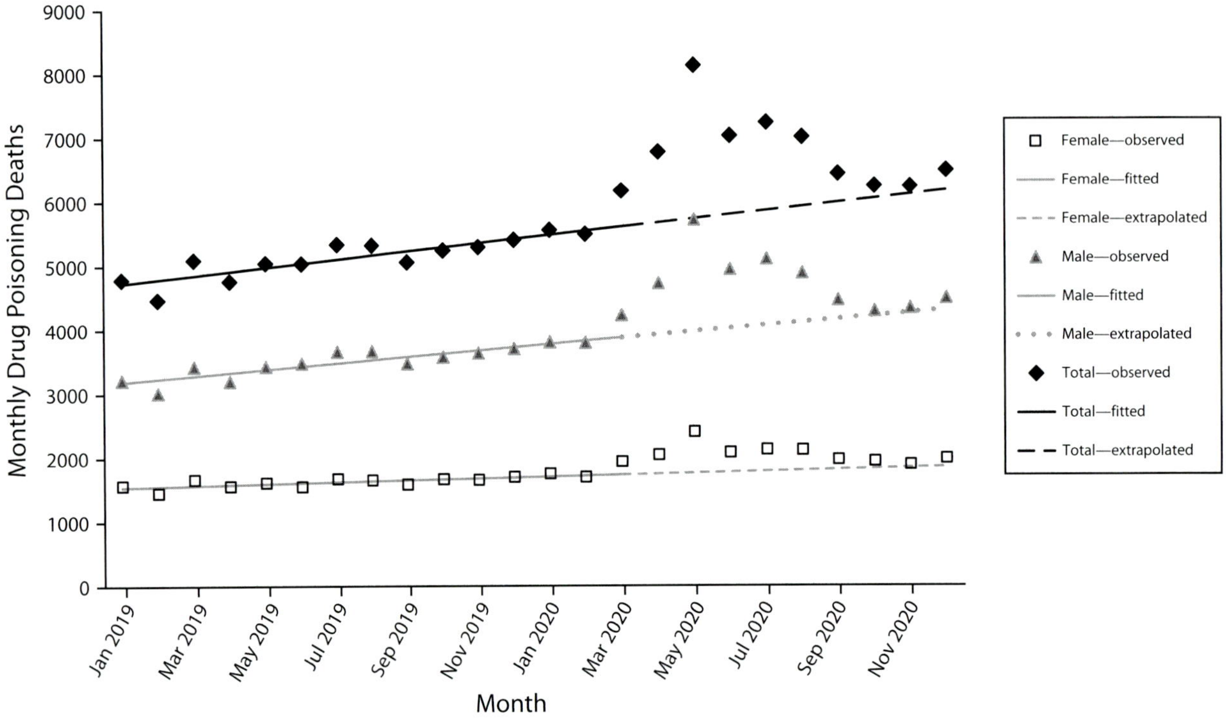

FIGURE 1— Monthly Drug-Poisoning Deaths Among Adults Aged 25–64 Years, by Sex and for Total Population: United States, 2019–2020

Note. Fitted lines are least-squares linear trend lines fitted to prepandemic counts; extrapolated lines are the continuation of the fitted lines during the pandemic months.

AJPH July 2024, Vol. 114, No. 7

of these additions altered the pattern of findings.

For our counterfactual analyses, we selected Iowa to exemplify the low SI, high ESI combination, whereas North Dakota, New York, and New Mexico represented the low SI, low ESI, high SI, high ESI, and high SI, low ESI combinations, respectively. The actual drug-poisoning death count for adults in the United States overall during April to December 2020 was 61 912. Results of our counterfactual simulations are presented graphically and numerically in Figure 2. If all states had followed the low SI, high ESI pattern, the United States would be predicted to have had 50 796 drug-poisoning deaths

TABLE 1— Relationship of COVID-19 Policy Interventions to Drug-Poisoning Mortality Among Adults Aged 25–64 Years, by Sex: United States, 2020

		Men				Women			
Model	Variable	IRR (95% CI)	Pseudo R^2	IR_0	IR_1	IRR (95% CI)	Pseudo R^2	IR_0	IR_1
1	SI	1.11 (1.06, 1.16)	0.67	1.52	1.68	1.09 (1.04, 1.14)	0.54	0.66	0.72
2	ESI	1.00 (0.98, 1.03)	0.67	1.50	1.51	0.99 (0.97, 1.02)	0.54	0.66	0.65
3	SI	1.15 (1.09, 1.20)	0.67	1.52	1.74	1.14 (1.09, 1.20)	0.54	0.66	0.75
3	ESI	0.97 (0.95, 1.00)	. . .	1.64	1.60	0.96 (0.93, 0.99)	. . .	0.72	0.69
4	SI	1.15 (1.09, 1.20)	0.67	1.52	1.74	1.14 (1.09, 1.20)	0.54	0.66	0.75
4	ESI	0.97 (0.95, 1.00)	. . .	1.64	1.60	0.96 (0.93, 0.99)	. . .	0.72	0.69

Note. CI = confidence interval; ESI = economic support index; IRR = incidence rate ratio; IR_0 = incidence rate, denominator of IRR; IR_1 = incidence rate, numerator of IRR; SI = stringency index. Regression includes controls for state–metro/nonmetro trends, area COVID-19 death rates, county-level poverty rates and political leanings, and month fixed effects.

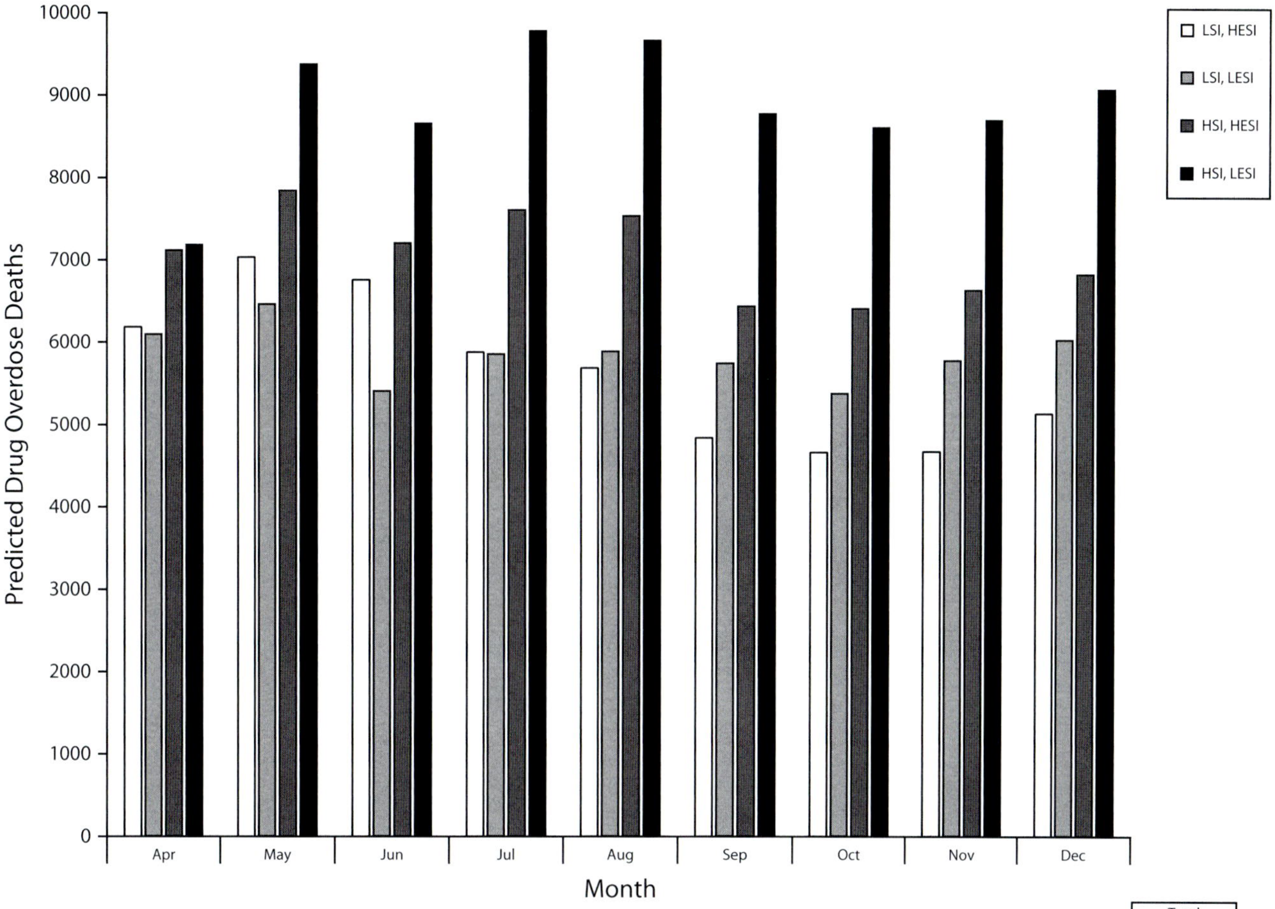

	Apr	May	Jun	Jul	Aug	Sep	Oct	Nov	Dec	Total
Actual	6 823	8 176	7 068	7 265	7 057	6 468	6 272	6 267	6 516	61 912
LSI, HESI	6 177	7 027	6 752	5 871	5 680	4 835	4 659	4 667	5 128	50 796
LSI, LESI	6 092	6 461	5 404	5 851	5 884	5 739	5 374	5 773	6 023	52 601
HSI, HESI	7 114	7 835	7 200	7 600	7 529	6 434	6 406	6 631	6 821	63 570
HSI, LESI	7 178	9 369	8 652	9 777	9 661	8 770	8 602	8 692	9 063	79 764

FIGURE 2— Predicted Drug-Poisoning Deaths Among Adults Aged 25–64 Years by Month as a Function of Counterfactual State SI and ESI Policies: United States, 2020

Note. ESI = economic support index; LSI/HSI = low/high stringency index; LESI/HESI = low/high economic support index; SI = stringency index.

(18% lower than actual). Our model predicted 52 601 deaths for the low SI, low ESI combination (15% lower than actual), 63 570 deaths for the high SI, high ESI combination (3% higher than actual), and 79 764 deaths for the high SI, low ESI combination (29% higher than actual).

DISCUSSION

To our knowledge, this study is the first to quantify the relation of states' COVID-19 policies that restricted in-person interaction and provided economic relief to drug overdose deaths among adults aged 25 to 64 years in 2020. We found that more extensive activity limitation policies predicted higher drug-poisoning mortality rates, whereas stronger economic relief policies predicted lower rates among both men and women.

Several previous studies found that stay-at-home orders predicted increases in drug overdose deaths among certain population subgroups in San Francisco, California[20]; Los Angeles County, California[22]; and Marion County, Indiana.[21] Although few studies have considered the effects of economic relief policies on population health outcomes during the COVID-19 pandemic, those that did focused on non–drug-related outcomes, finding that eviction moratoria were associated with better mental health[32] and lower rates of COVID-19 incidence and mortality.[33]

Our study extended this research in several ways. First, given that COVID-19 policies did not occur in isolation, it was important to examine multiple, often cooccurring policies. Our analysis advanced the literature by considering the whole United States rather than specific states or cities. Second, although several previous studies considered the effects of only stay-at-home orders on drug overdose deaths, our analysis considered multiple policies that restricted movement and in-person interactions along with those that provided economic relief.

Our study supports several important conclusions. First, although more robust activity limitation policies predicted increases in county-level drug-poisoning mortality, more robust economic support policies predicted decreases in county-level drug-poisoning mortality for both men and women. Stay-at-home orders, business and school closures, and gathering and travel restrictions may have contributed to higher rates of overdose because of demand-, supply-, and treatment-related factors, including isolation, boredom, loss of daily routine, poor mental health, ease of hiding drug use from others, solitary drug use, loss of employment, changes to the drug supply, and challenges in accessing treatment, recovery supports, and Naloxone.[7–12,33,35] The finding that policies that restricted in-person interaction were associated with larger increases in drug overdose deaths must be considered in a broader context of their potential reductions on COVID-19 mortality. Some evidence finds that state stringency policies predicted smaller increases in SARS-CoV-2 infections[36] and mortality rates in 2020.[37]

Second, economic support policies and activity limitation policies had countervailing associations with drug-poisoning deaths, but no state combined these policies in a way that predicted a decrease, or no increase, in such deaths. Strong economic support policies may have reduced stress among at-risk working-age adults by increasing their ability to pay bills and by reducing their risk of eviction. Studies that considered only the effects of stay-at-home orders specifically or activity limitations more generally without accounting for concomitant economic support policies may have overestimated the effects of stringency policies on drug overdose rates.

Finally, although no state enacted a combination of SI and ESI policies that fully offset each other in terms of drug-poisoning mortality, certain combinations predicted better outcomes than others. A combination of low stringency and high economic support predicted the smallest increases in drug-poisoning deaths, resulting in fewer deaths nationally than what actually occurred over the study period. Conversely, a combination of high stringency and low economic support predicted the largest increase, far exceeding the actual death count over the study period. These findings suggest that to reduce the risk of increasing overdose rates when governments enact restrictions on in-person activities, offsetting those actions with interventions that mitigate the adverse economic and social effects of such policies may be essential.

Limitations

Our study had some limitations. First, our conclusions rested on the untestable assumption that the extrapolated prepandemic trends in drug-poisoning mortality would have continued in the absence of the pandemic. The fact that observed overdose mortality for the United States overall and among counties on average closely followed the fitted prepandemic trend lines (Figure 1) supports this assumption.

Second, although states enacted various stringency policies, we do not know the extent to which individuals abided by them. However, previous research shows that state-level emergency declarations, social-distancing policies, and stay-at-home orders reduced human movement.[34,38]

Third, changes to the drug supply, including the increasing adulteration of nearly all classes of illicit drugs with fentanyl and the emergence of the highly fatal tranquilizer xylazine, might be a mechanism through which state policy changes could have influenced drug overdose trends. However, a lack of national data on drug supply precludes a determination of how changes in the supply of fentanyl, methamphetamine, and other drugs varied across the United States over this period. Our 2-stage estimation approach helped mitigate biases associated with not controlling for these factors.

Fourth, our analyses did not consider state drug policies. Policies that remained constant during the pandemic (e.g., Good Samaritan laws) would not influence our results because they are captured in the state fixed effects. Only a few states implemented new drug policies during the pandemic (e.g., telemedicine to initiate controlled substance prescriptions), but there was insufficient variation to control for these changes.

Fifth, death certificates may sometimes misclassify drug overdose deaths, and this misclassification may vary across geographic area.[39] However, to date, there is no evidence that misclassification of drug overdoses changed during the COVID-19 pandemic.

Finally, given that our research is ecological, we cannot determine the mechanisms through which policies might shape individuals' risk of overdose. For example, stringency policies may have been more detrimental to individuals who lived alone.

Public Health Implications

State policies to reduce SARS-CoV-2 spread and provide economic relief during 2020 may have had countervailing effects on drug mortality rates. Although activity limitation policies predicted higher drug-poisoning mortality rates, this was partly offset by economic relief policies. If the United States were to face another pandemic, policymakers should consider the potential negative externalities of policy decisions on other population health outcomes. Although policies that restricted in-person interaction may have reduced COVID-19 mortality rates,[37] results from our analyses suggest that they may have had the unintended consequence of increasing drug overdose deaths. AJPH

ABOUT THE AUTHORS

Douglas A. Wolf, Emily E. Wiemers, Yue Sun, and Jennifer Karas Montez are with the Aging Studies Institute, Syracuse University, Syracuse, NY. Shannon M. Monnat and Xue Zhang are with the Lerner Center for Public Health Promotion and Population Health, Syracuse University. Elyse R. Grossman is with the Epidemiology Research Branch, US National Institute on Drug Abuse, Gaithersburg, MD.

CORRESPONDENCE

Correspondence should be sent to Douglas A. Wolf, PhD, Aging Studies Institute, 314 Lyman Hall, Syracuse University, Syracuse, NY 13244 (e-mail: dawolf@syr.edu). Reprints can be ordered at http://www.ajph.org by clicking the "Reprints" link.

PUBLICATION INFORMATION

Full Citation: Wolf DA, Monnat SM, Wiemers EE, et al. State COVID-19 policies and drug overdose mortality among working-age adults in the United States, 2020. *Am J Public Health*. 2024;114(7): 714–722.

Acceptance Date: February 3, 2024.

DOI: https://doi.org/10.2105/AJPH.2024.307621

ORCID iDs:
Douglas A. Wolf https://orcid.org/0000-0002-4203-8993

Xue Zhang https://orcid.org/0000-0002-5786-4235

CONTRIBUTORS

D. A. Wolf, S. M. Monnat, Y. Sun, and X. Zhang prepared the data for analysis. D. A. Wolf and E. E. Wiemers designed and conducted the statistical analyses. S. M. Monnat provided overall project direction. All authors contributed to the writing and reviewed and approved the final version of the article.

ACKNOWLEDGMENTS

This project is funded by the National Institute on Drug Abuse (grant U01DA055972). The authors also acknowledge support from the National Institute on Aging (NIA)-funded Center for Aging and Policy Studies, Syracuse University (grant P30AG066583) and 2 research networks funded by the NIA (grants R24 AG065159 and 2R24 AG045061).

Note. The funders played no role in the writing of the article or the decision to submit it for publication. The views and opinions expressed in this article are those of the authors alone and do not necessarily represent the views, official policy, or position of the US Department of Health and Human Services or any of its affiliated institutions or agencies. E. R. Grossman was substantially involved in grant U01 DA055972, consistent with her role as a scientific officer.

CONFLICTS OF INTEREST

The authors have no conflicts of interest to report.

HUMAN PARTICIPANT PROTECTION

This study was reviewed by the institutional review board (IRB) at Syracuse University and deemed not to be human participant research (under 45 CFR 46.102(l)). IRB oversight and informed consent were not required.

REFERENCES

1. Centers for Disease Control and Prevention. National Vital Statistics System, mortality 2018–2021 on CDC WONDER online database. 2021. Available at: http://wonder.cdc.gov/ucd-icd10-expanded.html. Accessed April 9, 2023.
2. Monnat SM. Demographic and geographic variation in fatal drug overdoses in the United States, 1999–2020. *Ann Am Acad Pol Soc Sci*. 2023; 703(1):50–78. https://doi.org/10.1177/000271 62231154348
3. Spencer MR, Garnett FM, Miniño AM. Urban–rural differences in drug overdose death rates, 2020. *NCHS Data Brief*. 2022;(440):1–8. https://doi.org/10.15620/118601
4. Chiappini S, Guirguis A, John A, Corkery JM, Schifano F. COVID-19: the hidden impact on mental health and drug addiction. *Front Psychiatry*. 2020;11:767. https://doi.org/10.3389/fpsyt.2020.00767
5. Volkow ND. Collision of the COVID-19 and addiction epidemics. *Ann Intern Med*. 2020;173(1): 61–62. https://doi.org/10.7326/M20-1212
6. Barratt MJ, Aldridge J. No magic pocket: buying and selling on drug cryptomarkets in response to the COVID-19 pandemic and social restrictions. *Int J Drug Policy*. 2020;83:102894. https://doi.org/10.1016/j.drugpo.2020.102894
7. Gupta S, Montenovo L, Nguyen T, et al. Effects of social distancing policy on labor market outcomes. *Contemp Econ Policy*. 2023;41(1):166–193. https://doi.org/10.1111/coep.12582
8. Christie NC, Vojvodic V, Monterosso JR. The early impact of social distancing measures on drug use. *Subst Use Misuse*. 2021;56(7):997–1004. https://doi.org/10.1080/10826084.2021.1901934
9. Monnat S, Wheeler DC, Wiemers E, et al. States' COVID-19 physical distancing policies and working-age adult mental health outcomes. *Prev Med Rep*. 2023;35:102370. https://doi.org/10.1016/j.pmedr.2023.102370
10. Burns A, Albrecht K. Localized syndemic assemblages: COVID-19, substance use disorder, and overdose risk in small-town America. *RSF Russell Sage Found J Soc Sci*. 2022;8(8):245–262. https://doi.org/10.7758/RSF.2022.8.8.11
11. Dubey MJ, Ghosh R, Chatterjee S, Biswas P, Chatterjee S, Dubey S. COVID-19 and addiction. *Diabetes Metab Syndr*. 2020;14(5):817–823. https://doi.org/10.1016/j.dsx.2020.06.008
12. O'Donoghue AL, Biswas N, Dechen T, et al. Trends in filled naloxone prescriptions before and during the COVID-19 pandemic in the United States. *JAMA Health Forum*. 2021;2(5):e210393. https://doi.org/10.1001/jamahealthforum.2021.0393
13. Schlosser A, Harris S. Care during COVID-19: drug use, harm reduction, and intimacy during a global pandemic. *Int J Drug Policy*. 2020;83:102896. https://doi.org/10.1016/j.drugpo.2020.102896
14. Me A, Zeiler I, Garcia Yi J. COVID-19 and the drug supply chain: from production and trafficking to use. 2020. Available at: https://www.unodc.org/documents/data-and-analysis/covid/Covid-19-and-drug-supply-chain-Mai2020.pdf. Accessed December 18, 2023.
15. Alon T, Doepke M, Olmstead-Rumsey J, Tertilt M. *The Impact of COVID-19 on Gender Equality*. Cambridge, MA: National Bureau of Economic Research; 2020. NBER working paper 26947. https://doi.org/10.3386/w26947
16. Centers for Disease Control and Prevention. Racial and ethnic disparities in the prevalence of stress and worry, mental health conditions, and increased substance use among adults during the COVID-19 pandemic—United States, April and May 2020. *MMWR Morb Mortal Wkly Rep*. 2021;70(5):162–166. https://doi.org/10.15585/mmwr.mm7005a3
17. Mason M, Arukumar P, Feinglass J. The pandemic stay-at-home order and opioid-involved overdose fatalities. *JAMA*. 2021;325(24):2495–2496. https://doi.org/10.1001/jama.2021.6700
18. Root ED, Slavova S, LaRochelle M, et al. The impact of the national stay-at-home order on emergency department visits for suspected opioid overdose during the first wave of the COVID-19 pandemic. *Drug Alcohol Depend*. 2021;228: 108977. https://doi.org/10.1016/j.drugalcdep.2021.108977

19. Maeng D, Li Y, Lawrence M, et al. Impact of mandatory COVID-19 shelter-in-place order on controlled substance use among rural versus urban communities in the United States. *J Rural Health*. 2023;39(1):21–29. https://doi.org/10.1111/jrh.12688
20. Appa A, Rodda LN, Cawley C, et al. Drug overdose deaths before and after shelter-in-place orders during the COVID-19 pandemic in San Francisco. *JAMA Netw Open*. 2021;4(5):e2110452. https://doi.org/10.1001/jamanetworkopen.2021.10452
21. Glober N, Mohler G, Huynh P, et al. Impact of COVID-19 pandemic on drug overdoses in Indianapolis. *J Urban Health*. 2020;97(6):802–807. https://doi.org/10.1007/s11524-020-00484-0
22. Kelley MA, Lucas J, Stewart E, Goldman D, Doctor JN. Opioid-related deaths before and after COVID-19 stay-at-home orders in Los Angeles County. *Drug Alcohol Depend*. 2021;228:109028. https://doi.org/10.1016/j.drugalcdep.2021.109028
23. Ali F, Russell C, Nafeh F, Rehm J, LeBlanc S, Elton-Marshall T. Changes in substance supply and use characteristics among people who use drugs (PWUD) during the COVID-19 global pandemic: a national qualitative assessment in Canada. *Int J Drug Policy*. 2021;93:103237. https://doi.org/10.1016/j.drugpo.2021.103237
24. Centers for Disease Control and Prevention. US census populations with bridged race categories. October 28, 2022. Available at: https://www.cdc.gov/nchs/nvss/bridged_race.htm. Accessed August 20, 2022.
25. Hale T, Angrist N, Goldszmidt R, et al. A global panel database of pandemic policies (Oxford COVID-19 Government Response Tracker). *Nat Hum Behav*. 2021;5(4):529–538. https://doi.org/10.1038/s41562-021-01079-8
26. Platt E, Moran-McCabe K, Cook A, Burris S. Trends in US state public health emergency laws, 2021–2022. *Am J Public Health*. 2023;113(3):288–296. https://doi.org/10.2105/AJPH.2022.307214
27. Hamad R, Lyman KA, Lin F, et al. The US COVID-19 county policy database: a novel resource to support pandemic-related research. *BMC Public Health*. 2022;1882(1):1882. https://doi.org/10.1186/s12889-022-14132-6
28. Zhang X, Warner ME, Meredity G. Factors limiting US public health emergency authority during COVID-19. *Int J Health Plann Manage*. 2023;38(5):1569–1582. https://doi.org/10.1002/hpm.3694
29. US Department of Agriculture. Rural–urban continuum codes. 2020. Available at: https://www.ers.usda.gov/data-products/rural-urban-continuum-codes.aspx. Accessed May 5, 2021.
30. Shadish WR, Cook TD, Campbell DT. *Experimental and Quasi-Experimental Designs for Generalized Causal Inference*. Boston, MA: Houghton Mifflin; 2002.
31. Gourieroux C, Monfort A, Trognon A. Pseudo maximum likelihood methods: applications to Poisson models. *Econometrica*. 1984;52(3):701–720. https://doi.org/10.2307/1913472
32. Borusyak K, Jaravel X, Spiess J. Revisiting event study designs: robust and efficient estimation. *arXiv*. 2022:2108.12419. https://doi.org/10.48550/arXiv.2108.12419
33. Courtemanche C, Garuccio J, Le A, Pinkston J, Yelowitz A. Strong social distancing measures in the United States reduced the COVID-19 growth rate. *Hum Aff (Millwood)*. 2020;39(7):1237–1246. https://doi.org/10.4324/9781003141402-20
34. Leifheit KM, Pollack CE, Raifman J, et al. Variation in state-level eviction moratorium protections and mental health among US adults during the COVID-19 pandemic. *JAMA Netw Open*. 2021;4(12):e2139585. https://doi.org/10.1001/jamanetworkopen.2021.39585
35. Fowler JH, Hill SJ, Levin R, Obradovich N. Stay-at-home orders associate with subsequent decreases in COVID-19 cases and fatalities in the United States. *PLoS One*. 2021;16(6):e0248849. https://doi.org/10.1371/journal.pone.0248849
36. Bollyky TJ, Castro E, Aravkin AY, et al. Assessing COVID-19 pandemic policies and behaviours and their economic and educational trade-offs across US states from Jan 1, 2020, to July 31, 2022: an observational analysis. *Lancet*. 2023;401(10385):1341–1360. https://doi.org/10.1016/S0140-6736(23)00461-0
37. Sun Y, Bisesti EM. Political economy of the COVID-19 pandemic: how state policies shape county-level disparities in COVID-19 deaths. *Socius*. 2023;9:23780231221149902. https://doi.org/10.1177/23780231221149902
38. Leifheit KM, Linton SL, Raifman J, et al. Expiring eviction moratoriums and COVID-19 incidence and mortality. *Am J Epidemiol*. 2021;190(12):2503–2510. https://doi.org/10.1093/aje/kwab196
39. Ruhm CJ. Geographic variation in opioid and heroin involved drug poisoning mortality rates. *Am J Prev Med*. 2017;53(6):745–753. https://doi.org/10.1016/j.amepre.2017.06.009

Convivial Populations: Ivan Illich and Public Health in the 21st Century

Aldis H. Petriceks, MPH

Ivan Illich (1926–2002) was a historian, social critic, and professor at multiple universities. He came to intellectual fame through his criticisms of modern institutions, including health care, and his concern with social structures that he believed to impede human flourishing. However, Illich has not been thoroughly explored as a source of insight for public health professionals. Although he populates the medical and public health literature, discourse remains sparse about how Illich might contribute to key conversations in public health today. In this article, I explore Illich's potential contributions to modern public health through one of his seminal works, *Tools for Conviviality*. I frame Illich as a valuable conversational partner for public health professionals at a crucial moment in the field's history. (*Am J Public Health*. 2024;114(7):723–728. https://doi.org/10.2105/AJPH.2024.307675)

AJPH July 2024, Vol. 114, No. 7

Today, the writer Ivan Illich is often remembered as a polemicist who criticized major institutions. "The medical establishment has become a major threat to health," he wrote in *Medical Nemesis* (later updated as *Limits to Medicine*), which remains perhaps his best-known work.[1(p19)] His characterization as a critic of modern health care was earned through that book, in which he argued that society had "transferred to physicians the exclusive right to determine what constitutes sickness, who is or might become sick, and what shall be done to such people."[1(p21)] Yet Illich was not simply a polemicist of modern medicine, and his interests and purposes went far beyond the critique of health care. He reflected deeply on, and largely praised, the activities and advances of public health in the 20th century, and engaged with social and ethical questions that continue to define the field decades after his death. However, he has received little attention for his relevance to modern public health.

In this article, I reexamine Illich's intellectual legacy for public health. I argue that Illich's concerns about health and society go beyond clinical medicine and medicalization, and provide important insights into contemporary public health practice. His critique of the "disembodying" aspects of modern society—in which risk determines individual behavior and solutions are sought in impersonal institutions—can be (and has been) used to undermine public health measures, but it may also guide public health toward new, more thoughtful approaches in an increasingly complex world and society. To highlight this potential positive contribution, I examine not the better-known *Limits to Medicine* but *Tools for Conviviality*—an earlier, shorter, and more general book that demonstrates and contextualizes Illich's wide-ranging concerns for modern society.

ILLICH IN CONTEXT

Ivan Illich was born in 1926, in Vienna, Austria. He was ordained as a priest in the Roman Catholic church after undergraduate studies in histology and crystallography, and graduate work in history.[2] Frustrated with Catholic bureaucracy, Illich left Rome to conduct research on medieval history at Princeton University in 1951, but while passing through New York City he grew enamored with the plight of Puerto Rican immigrants and became a parish priest in the heavily Puerto Rican community of Washington Heights. He spent five years there before moving to Puerto Rico to become vice rector of the Catholic University at Ponce.

Illich remained on the island for another five years, until his resistance to the political involvement of Catholic bishops in Puerto Rico led to his removal from the diocese.[2] He later suspended his priestly duties in the 1960s, partly in response to disagreements with Catholic hierarchy, and devoted himself to writing and teaching.[2] In turn, the 1970s and early 1980s marked the height of his activity as a writer and public intellectual, and saw the publication of *Tools for Conviviality* (1973) as well as *Limits to Medicine* (1976). For Illich, these books were a response to what he saw as the institutional overmanagement of the lives of individuals and communities, and an attempt to focus attention on the social conditions that would promote healthy, autonomous flourishing in modern life. They are not always portrayed in this light. The *New York Times* wrote in its 1976 review of *Limits to Medicine* that from Illich's "cocoon of apparent radical humanism there ultimately emerges no bright butterfly of revolutionary change but rather . . . a caterpillar of petty conservatism"[3]; although later critics would recognize the prescience in many of Illich's diagnoses, he remains a polemical figure for many in modern medicine.[3–5]

TOOLS FOR CONVIVIALITY

However, *Tools for Conviviality* remains a less explored book in the health professions, not least in public health. In this work, Illich outlines his critique of institutions as diverse as health care, school systems, transport, and energy distribution, opening with a brief glance at the history of public health and medicine in the 20th century. This history is framed by two "watersheds," beyond which the professions progressively passed. The first watershed is defined largely by improvements in communal resources—clean water, sanitation, agricultural developments—that fall within the purview of public health. The second watershed is defined by expanded institutional power to manage individual health and behavior, through the activities of clinical as well as public health authorities.

Illich argues that an unlimited appetite for technological expansion and institutional management has much to do with the difference between these two watersheds. According to this argument, the first watershed arose through the employment of technology and public health knowledge, oriented toward the healthy use of resources by individuals and communities; the second watershed arose through overexpansion of clinical and public health activities, oriented toward the protection and prolongation of human life. As philosopher Carl Mitcham writes, *Tools for Conviviality* becomes, in this context, a reflection on "how to avoid or respond to the second threshold, after which technology begins to be less unambiguously effective in meeting basic human needs."[6(p46)]

"The year 1913," Illich writes in the opening pages of the book, "marks a watershed in the history of modern medicine."[7(p13)] Around this time, "a patient began to have more than a fifty-fifty chance that a graduate of a medical school would provide him with a specifically effective treatment," supposing that such a treatment existed for a known disease.[7(p13)] This watershed bore witness to reductions in infant mortality, revolutions in the treatment of infectious diseases, and effective crisis management. Morbidity and mortality plunged, owing largely "to changes in sanitation, agriculture, marketing, and general attitudes toward life."[7(p13)] Moreover, these improvements were measurable and quantifiable:

> Germ-free water reduced infant mortality due to diarrhea, aspirin reduced the pain of rheumatism, and malaria could be controlled by quinine. . . . People began to understand the relationship between health and a balanced diet, fresh air, calisthenics, pure water and soap. New devices ranging from toothbrushes to Band-Aids and condoms became widely available. The positive contribution of modern medicine to individual health during the early part of the twentieth century can hardly be questioned.[7(p18)]

The second watershed occurred in approximately the mid-1950s, when the "monopoly of the medical profession was extended" beyond the protection of safe, common resources for health, and "over an increasing range of everyday occurrences in every man's life."[7(p14)] According to Illich, the deleterious effects of this "radical monopoly" are visible in heightened costs of both prevention and treatment, overpopulation, the medicalization of death, social biases in medical practice and research, and the irresponsible prescription of medication. Increasingly costly measures to extend or improve life mask the "malignant expansion of *institutional* health care which is at the root of the rising costs and demands and the decline in well-being" of modern populations.[7(p18)] This decline may be difficult to quantify, but that is part of the argument: "Society can have no quantitative standards by which to add up the negative value of illusion, social control, prolonged suffering, loneliness, genetic deterioration, and frustration" brought about by medicalization.[7(p19)]

Clearly, Illich's reputation as antimedical polemicist is not entirely unearned. But for all that has been written—even in support—of this analysis of the second watershed, later discourse on Illich has at times omitted his attention to the first watershed. Although Illich was certainly concerned about the medicalization of society and about industrialized health care, his concern originated in a deep attention to personal autonomy, social solidarity, and the social conditions conducive to healthy lifestyles. This concern is manifest in his reflection on what he calls the "crisis of medicine":

> [The crisis of medicine] results from the development of a professional complex supported and exhorted by society to provide increasingly "better" health, and from the willingness of clients to serve as guinea pigs in this vain experiment. People have lost the right to declare themselves sick; society now accepts their claims to sickness only after certification by medical bureaucrats.[7(p18)]

His concern was that health was no longer an activity that people pursued—an activity that could be enriched and enabled by medical care and public health endeavors—but a product that people received from impersonal institutions. In the future that he predicted, people would treat genetic risk as concrete reality, public health authorities would restrict movement and activity based on abstract statistical constructs, and doctors would promote complicated treatments requiring ever-increasing specialization and regulation. In this future, individuals and their communities would lose not only a degree of personal health autonomy but also a sense of responsibility for those aspects of daily life that brought medicine and public health to the first watershed. If people came to see health simply as a product to be received from doctors and defined by public health experts, society itself would become sick.

Illich's response to the institutional overmanagement of health was not (as he is sometimes caricatured) to return to a lost world of self-care and self-sustenance devoid of high technology. His vision was rather to incorporate the advancements of technological society within the structural and conceptual developments of the first watershed. Broadly, this vision was united by his concept of conviviality, which he defined as "individual freedom realized in personal interdependence," as opposed to "the conditioned response of persons to the demands made upon them by others, and by a man-made environment."[7(p24)] In turn, a convivial society would be the result of "social arrangements that guarantee for each member the most ample and free access to the tools of the community and limit this freedom only in favor of another member's equal freedom."[7(p25)]

INSIGHTS AND IMPLICATIONS OF *TOOLS FOR CONVIVIALITY*

This vision has several potential meanings for public health in the United States. Most basically, it suggests that Illich is an ambiguous but valuable voice for public health professionals, who have long struggled under insufficient funding despite increasing health care spending over the past several decades.[8] As an unexpected voice of support for public health, Illich argues that excessive and monolithic attention to health care inhibits human flourishing through diminished attention not only to social conditions, but also to human autonomy and subsistence. Such arguments were in line with his broader, ongoing efforts to galvanize those "who struggle to preserve the biosphere, and those who oppose a style of life characterized by a monopoly of commodities over activities . . . to recover and enlarge in some way *the commons*."[9(p36)] By "commons," Illich meant "an aspect of the environment that was limited, necessary for different groups in different ways, but which, in a strictly economic sense, was not perceived as scarce,"[2(p220)] a meaning not wholly removed from what we mean today when we describe the social determinants of health.

But despite Illich's perhaps surprising support for much of public health, his emphasis on autonomy also contains the seed of his ambiguity for the profession. He viewed vaccines as convivial tools but was against vaccine mandates, and his arguments against institutional overmanagement can be taken as resistance to some of the most basic activities of modern public health, such as those involved in the control of infectious disease. Indeed, the COVID-19 pandemic has provided at least one example of Illich's ideas being used in a potentially dangerous manner. During the early months of the pandemic, Giorgio Agamben, a renowned Italian philosopher highly influenced by Illich, wrote that public health measures to contain the virus had been "frenetic, irrational, and entirely unfounded," and suggested that citizens who willingly followed these measures had suffered incredible damage to their human condition "solely in the name of a risk that it was not possible to specify."[10] This inherent skepticism of risk and institutional management has deep connections to Illich's work, in which statistical constructs are sometimes depicted as disembodying practices that remove human decision-making from the here-and-now of everyday life and place it in the hands of technocratic experts.[11] This is likely one aspect of Illich's legacy that makes him a complicated figure in public health today. On the one hand, such skepticism and diversity of opinion is necessary for a functioning democracy and public health system, and may indeed carry important criticism for public health practices. But taken too far in the other direction, hardened dissent can serve largely to breed distrust in an already fragile social and political order.

Yet there is an even more important contribution to public health that comes through in *Tools for Conviviality*, and this lies in the definition of conviviality, the "individual freedom realized in personal interdependence" spoken of earlier. Much of Illich's critique of modern institutions had to do with their distance from the people whose activities and lives they were regulating. Mass obligatory schooling drew his criticism because it took little account of the unique needs and skills of each individual. Highway systems did the same because they inhibited free movement while purporting to create it. To the extent that public health receives similar critique in Illich's work, this criticism relates to restrictive policies enacted on communities who have little input in the matter. For Illich, "individual freedom realized in personal interdependence" suggests that a convivial public health is indeed possible, but that it must involve genuine contact, exchange, and interdependence between public health professionals and the communities that they aim to serve.

At its core, this implies a healthy dose of community engagement and community input on potential public health policies, which sounds unambiguously positive but is, of course, highly complex in practice, as the COVID-19 pandemic also demonstrated when numerous communities pushed back against pandemic measures.[12–14] Public health officials may engage the public all they want on issues of masking, isolation, or vaccine mandates, but they will need to decide what actions to recommend or enforce, and these may ultimately run counter to the desires of a community, or many communities, or select portions of communities.[15] In such situations, Illich does indeed fail to produce the bright butterfly of a revolutionary idea. Yet as public health ethicists continue to debate the proper balance between autonomy and the public good in the setting of such conflicts, it is valuable to recall that for Illich, the core principle in this debate was not one of ethics but of friendship and interpersonal care.[11,16–18] For him, health could never simply be about "saving lives" or "eliminating disease," but rather the art of living and dying well, which included a humility toward the unknown and an awareness of death. What this means in practice is of course uncertain, but Illich's ideas may contribute to a culture in which public health is seen, even in this socially polarized moment, as a convivial form of interpersonal care, rather than an impersonal institution organized to provide and protect a thing called health.

Robert Dingwall, a sociologist, made an argument along these lines recently in the *BMJ*.[19] In his brief article, "More to Illich Than Overtreatment," published in 2022, Dingwall argued that Illich's critique of clinical medicine—often taken as the thesis of *Limits to Medicine*—was in fact secondary to his broader social critiques that appeared in books such as *Tools for Conviviality*. For Dingwall, the deeper problem that Illich recognized was "the way in which biomedicine had promoted the idea that a good society was defined purely by the health of its people in terms defined largely by the medical profession."[19] The author found evidence for this problem "in the ways in which the collateral societal harms of pandemic management have been dismissed as unworthy of consideration, and the cult of zero infection has skewed debates over non-pharmaceutical interventions and childhood vaccination."[19] In this light, he argued that Illich remains valuable for his concern with balance and proportion, and for his recognition that human beings exist in a relationship—not a war—with illness and death: "[T]he questions that [Illich] asked have taken on a new relevance as we reflect on what went right and wrong with pandemic management," Dingwall wrote, suggesting that this was ample reason "to revive interest in [Illich's] work."[19]

This sensitivity to difficult questions has perhaps never been so important. Over the past several decades, trust in US government institutions has diminished, and this distrust has worsened since the onset of the COVID-19 pandemic.[20–22] As James Hamblin, a journalist and lecturer at the Yale School of Public Health, wrote in the *New York Times*, "69 percent of Americans believed what they heard from [the Centers for Disease Control and Prevention]" at the beginning of the pandemic, but by early 2022 "that [had] fallen to 44 percent."[22] One possible interpretation of this decline, Hamblin wrote, "is that politics and science have melded so completely that the result has been neither scientifically nor politically effective."[22] This is an almost Illichian statement, encouraging public health professionals to recognize the inherently social nature of their policies and to distinguish between those policies and the science behind them. Such transparency about the values

AJPH July 2024, Vol. 114, No. 7

and political considerations that influence our decision-making may promote greater trust, effectiveness, and equity in public health.[14,22,23] As Hamblin noted:

> Trust in a system does not mean always agreeing that the correct decision has been made but that decisions were made in good faith, transparently, taking all perspectives into account. We haven't had enough of this in the pandemic.[22]

One of Illich's most timely traits was his attempt to distinguish science from political decision-making and thus to promote a synergy, as opposed to a blurring, between the two.

CONCLUSION

Illich was not correct in all his social diagnoses, and no one will mistake him for a mastermind of public health policy. But he was deeply attentive to the importance of human activity and relationship for the health and flourishing of communities, and from this attention radiates his several (and at times ambiguous) meanings for public health. On the one hand, he is an unexpected voice of support, with a rich intellectual background and skill set, for the importance of public health as an enhancement of the commons. Paired with his criticisms of excessive medical spending and medicalization, works like *Tools for Conviviality* provide forceful arguments for strong systems to ensure that individuals and communities create the social conditions that will enable them to flourish autonomously and convivially. At the same time, his consistent emphasis on autonomy and his stance against institutional management raise challenging dissent for public health officials tasked with restricting autonomy for the public good. But even in the face of this dissent, Illich centers his work on a reverence for friendship, personal interdependence, and human contact, which may aid public health in the United States as it navigates a cultural moment of social polarization and diminished trust in major institutions.

Such contributions may not qualify Illich as a prophet of public health in the same way that he became the "Prophet of Cuernavaca" for his social and intellectual activities in Latin America.[24] But like the Old Testament prophets he revered, Illich was always more a visionary than a manager, and this makes him no less important as a voice in the desert. AJPH

ABOUT THE AUTHOR

Aldis H. Petriceks is with Harvard Medical School, Boston, MA, and the Columbia University Mailman School of Public Health, New York, NY.

CORRESPONDENCE

Correspondence should be sent to Aldis H. Petriceks, 107 Avenue Louis Pasteur, Boston, MA 02115 (e-mail: aldis_petriceks@hms.harvard.edu). Reprints can be ordered at http://www.ajph.org by clicking the "Reprints" link.

PUBLICATION INFORMATION

Full Citation: Petriceks AH. Convivial populations: Ivan Illich and public health in the 21st century. *Am J Public Health*. 2024;114(7):723–728.

Acceptance Date: March 25, 2024.

DOI: https://doi.org/10.2105/AJPH.2024.307675

ACKNOWLEDGMENTS

I am grateful to Ron Bayer, PhD, for his insightful commentary on this manuscript, and for his generous mentorship. I also thank my mentors in the General Public Health program at the Columbia University Mailman School of Public Health, for their support of this work.

CONFLICTS OF INTEREST

There are no conflicts of interest to disclose.

REFERENCES

1. Illich I. *Limits to Medicine*. London, UK: Marion Boyars Publishers; 1976.
2. Cayley D. *Ivan Illich: An Intellectual Journey*. University Park, PA: Pennsylvania State University Press; 2021. https://doi.org/10.1515/9780271089140
3. Geiger JA. Medical nemesis. *New York Times*. May 2, 1976. Available at: https://www.nytimes.com/1976/05/02/archives/medical-nemesis-the-20thcenturys-leading-luddite-turns-to-medicine.html. Accessed March 1, 2024.
4. O'Mahony S. Medical nemesis 40 years on: the enduring legacy of Ivan Illich. *J R Coll Physicians Edinb*. 2016;46(2):134–139. https://doi.org/10.4997/jrcpe.2016.214
5. Thomas L. Rx for Illich. *New York Rev Books*. September 1976. Available at: https://www.nybooks.com/articles/1976/09/16/rx-for-illich. Accessed November 22, 2023.
6. Mitcham C. Tools for conviviality: argument, insight, influence. *Conspiratio*. 2023;(5):41–92. Available at: https://thinkingafterivanillich.net/wp-content/uploads/2022/10/Tools-for-Conviviality-Argument-Insight-Influence.pdf. Accessed February 2, 2024.
7. Illich I. *Tools for Conviviality*. London, UK: Marion Boyars Publishers; 1973.
8. Alfonso YN, Leider JP, Resnick B, McCullough J Mac, Bishai D. US public health neglected: flat or declining spending left states ill equipped to respond to COVID-19. *Health Aff (Millwood)*. 2021;40(4):664–671. https://doi.org/10.1377/hlthaff.2020.01084
9. Illich I. *Gender*. London, UK: Marion Boyars Publishers; 1982.
10. Kotsko A. What happened to Giorgio Agamben? *Slate*. February 2022. Available at: https://slate.com/human-interest/2022/02/giorgio-agamben-covid-holocaust-comparison-right-wing-protest.html. Accessed February 23, 2024.
11. Illich I. *In the Mirror of the Past*. London, UK: Marion Boyars Publishers; 1991.
12. Wallace-Wells D. Dr. Fauci looks back: "something clearly went wrong." *New York Times*. April 24, 2023. Available at: https://www.nytimes.com/interactive/2023/04/24/magazine/dr-fauci-pandemic.html. Accessed February 21, 2024.
13. Bardosh K, De Figueiredo A, Gur-Arie R, et al. The unintended consequences of COVID-19 vaccine policy: why mandates, passports and restrictions may cause more harm than good. *BMJ Glob Health*. 2022;7(5):1–14. https://doi.org/10.1136/bmjgh-2022-008684
14. Lowe AE, Voo TC, Lee LM, et al. Uncertainty, scarcity and transparency: public health ethics and risk communication in a pandemic. *Lancet Reg Health Am*. 2022;16:100374. https://doi.org/10.1016/j.lana.2022.100374
15. Fairchild AL, Bayer R. Why using fear to promote COVID-19 vaccination and mask wearing could backfire. The Conversation. 2021. Available at: https://theconversation.com/why-using-fear-to-promote-covid-19-vaccination-and-mask-wearing-could-backfire-153865. Accessed February 22, 2023.
16. Colgrove J, Bayer R. Manifold restraints: liberty, public health, and the legacy of Jacobson v Massachusetts. *Am J Public Health*. 2005;95(4):571–576. https://doi.org/10.2105/AJPH.2004.055145

17. Bayer R. The continuing tensions between individual rights and public health. *EMBO Rep.* 2007; 8(12):1099–1103. https://doi.org/10.1038/sj.embor.7401134
18. Bayer R, Fairchild AL. The genesis of public health ethics. *Bioethics.* 2004;18(6):473–492. https://doi.org/10.1111/j.1467-8519.2004.00412.x
19. Dingwall R. More to Illich than overtreatment: his work is relevant as we reflect on pandemic management. *BMJ.* 2022;378:o1716. https://doi.org/10.1136/bmj.o1716
20. SteelFisher GK, Findling MG, Caporello HL, et al. Trust in US federal, state, and local public health agencies during COVID-19: responses and policy implications. *Health Aff (Millwood).* 2023;42(3): 328–337. https://doi.org/10.1377/hlthaff.2022.01204
21. Blendon RJ, Benson JM. Trust in medicine, the health system & public health. *Daedalus.* 2022;151(4):67–82. https://doi.org/10.1162/daed_a_01944
22. Hamblin J. Can public health be saved? *New York Times.* March 12, 2022. Available at: https://www.nytimes.com/2022/03/12/opinion/public-health-trust.html. Accessed February 22, 2023.
23. Mello MM, Gostin LO. Public health law modernization 2.0: rebalancing public health powers and individual liberty in the age of COVID-19. *Health Aff (Millwood).* 2023;42(3):318–327. https://doi.org/10.1377/hlthaff.2022.01292
24. Hartch T. *The Prophet of Cuernavaca: Ivan Illich and the Crisis of the West.* New York, NY: Oxford University Press; 2015. https://doi.org/10.1093/acprof:oso/9780190204563.001.0001

Black Americans' Drug Mortality Increases and Local Employment Opportunities, 2010–2021

Sehun Oh, PhD, and Manuel Cano, PhD

Objectives. To test the associations between local employment opportunities for the Black workforce and drug mortality among Black Americans, while examining the potential moderating effects of fentanyl seizure rates.

Methods. We derived data from the National Center for Health Statistics' restricted-access Multiple Cause of Death file, linked with county-level job counts, drug supply, and other characteristics from the US Census Bureau and the Centers for Disease Control and Prevention. After examining the characteristics of counties by the magnitudes of increases in drug mortality from 2010–2013 to 2018–2021, we conducted a first-differenced regression analysis to test the associations between the job-to-Black workforce ratio and age-adjusted drug mortality rates among Black Americans in US counties and test the moderating effects of state-level fentanyl seizure rates.

Results. One more job per 100 Black workers was associated with 0.29 fewer drug overdose deaths per 100 000 Black Americans in the county. This negative association was stronger in the counties of the states with higher increases in fentanyl seizure rates.

Conclusions. Increasing employment opportunities can be an important strategy for preventing Black Americans' drug mortality, especially among those living in areas with higher increases in fentanyl seizure rates. (*Am J Public Health*. 2024;114(7):729–732. https://doi.org/10.2105/AJPH.2024.307646)

AJPH July 2024, Vol. 114, No. 7

After a decade of outpacing growth in drug mortality, Black Americans surpassed White Americans' drug mortality rates in 2020.[1] This trend coincides with the beginning of the third phase of the US drug epidemic, primarily driven by synthetic opioids, including illicitly manufactured fentanyl.[2] The literature on social determinants of health emphasizes the role of "deep-seated inequalities in living conditions," such as employment, to better understand the newly emerging drug epidemic pattern.[3] Research shows that disconnection from the workforce creates collective frustration and hopelessness, family disintegration, and community violence and crime, increasing drug use as a refuge from psychological distress.[2,4] In particular, illicitly manufactured fentanyl is mostly street-supplied[5] and disproportionately affects individuals in communities lacking employment opportunities, especially among Black populations.[3]

Despite the potential contribution of local employment contexts to Black Americans' drug mortality increases during the 2010s, few studies have investigated this relationship. The present study aims to examine the associations between employment opportunities for the Black workforce and drug mortality among Black Americans throughout the 2010s, while also examining the role of an increased supply of fentanyl, which drives the emerging drug epidemic. Specifically, we linked administrative data on county-level drug mortality and job counts to estimate the associations between the job-to-Black workforce ratio and the Black population's drug mortality rates in US counties and the moderating effects of state-level fentanyl seizure rates.

METHODS

We drew county-level drug mortality data from the National Center for Health Statistics' restricted-access Multiple Cause of Death file, a compilation of death certificate data from US Vital Statistics jurisdictions. Drug-involved overdose deaths of any intent were identified according to the *International Classification of Diseases, 10th Revision* (Geneva, Switzerland: World Health Organization; 1992) codes X40–X44 (unintentional drug poisoning), X60–X64 (intentional drug poisoning), X85 (drug poisoning homicide), or Y10–Y14 (drug poisoning of undetermined intent). For reliable estimation of drug mortality rates among non-Hispanic Black individuals, we pooled 4 years of mortality data (2010–2013 and 2018–2021). Then we linked the data with statistics on county-level job counts and drug supply (including state-level fentanyl seizures from the US Drug Enforcement Administration) as well as sociodemographic data from the US Census Longitudinal Employer-Household Dynamics Origin-Destination Employment Statistics, opioid prescribing rate map files from the Centers for Disease Control and Prevention (CDC), and American Community Surveys. Given the CDC's suppression of subnational rates with fewer than 10 deaths, our analytic sample was restricted to 214 counties with at least 10 deaths among Black residents in 2010–2013 and 2018–2021, predominantly metropolitan counties with a larger Black population (Appendix Table A, available as a supplement to the online version of this article at https://ajph.org).

Measures

We examined the following measures from 2010–2013 and 2018–2021 and computed the first differences (value in 2018–2021 minus value in 2010–2013) for our first-differenced regression models. The outcome variable was each county's age-adjusted drug overdose mortality rate per 100 000 Black residents. The independent variable was a county's number of jobs occupied by Black workers divided by the county's number of Black individuals aged 18 to 64 years. As a moderator, we examined the rate of state-level fentanyl or fentanyl analog seizures per 100 000 population. County-level sociodemographic and drug-supply controls included percentage Black population, percentage males, percentage individuals aged 65 years and older, percentage individuals aged 25 years and older without a high-school diploma, percentage veterans, percentage vacant housing, percentage unemployed individuals, median household income, region (Midwest, Northeast, South, West), and opioid prescribing rates.

Analyses

We conducted the statistical analyses in 3 steps. First, we examined the characteristics of counties with varying magnitudes of drug mortality increases among Black residents from 2010–2013 to 2018–2021. Second, we estimated first-differenced regression models to test the associations between the job-to-Black workforce ratio and age-adjusted drug mortality rates among the Black population and its interaction with state-level fentanyl seizure rates. Our first-differenced regression models removed time-constant unobserved confounders at the county level, allowing for more accurate estimation. Lastly, we estimated Black Americans' drug mortality rates across the job-to-Black workforce ratios, separately for the counties in the states with varying levels of change in fentanyl seizure rates.

RESULTS

The increases in the drug mortality rate among the Black population from 2010–2013 to 2018–2021 were not uniformly observed across the counties, ranging from −0.7 to 110.7 per 100 000 population, with a mean increase of 27.5. As presented in Appendix Table B, the top-tercile group—primarily Midwest and Northeast counties with a lower median household income—reported a mean increase of 48.7 deaths per 100 000, signifying a 327% increase. On the other hand, the bottom-tercile group—mostly Southern counties with higher median household income—had a mean increase of 10.6 deaths per 100 000, a 115% increase.

When we adjusted for state-level fentanyl seizure rates and county-level controls (model 2), 1 more job per 100 Black workers was associated with 0.29 fewer drug overdose deaths per 100 000 Black population (see Table 1). Model 3 shows the statistically significant moderating effect of the state fentanyl seizure rates ($b = -0.01$; $P < .001$), implying that the negative associations between the job-to-Black workforce ratio and Black Americans' drug-related mortality were stronger in counties with higher fentanyl seizure rates. For the counties in the highest tercile of fentanyl seizure rate growths, for instance, the magnitudes of increases in drug mortality for having 50 fewer and 50 more jobs (per 100 Black workers) in 2018 to 2021 compared with 2010 to 2013 were 98.6 and 4.9 per 100 000 Black population, respectively (Appendix Figure A). On the other hand, these relationships were nonexistent in the counties of states in the lowest tercile of the fentanyl seizure rate increases.

TABLE 1— Associations Between Job Opportunities and the Age-Adjusted Drug Overdose Mortality Rates Among Non-Hispanic Black Populations by First-Difference Regression Model: US Counties, 2010–2013 and 2018–2021

	Model 1		Model 2		Model 3	
Sociodemographic Characteristic	**b (SE)**	**B (SE)**	**b (SE)**	**B (SE)**	**b (SE)**	**B (SE)**
Independent variable and moderator						
Difference in jobs per 100 Black workers	−0.22 (0.14)	−0.11 (0.08)	−0.29* (0.14)	−0.15* (0.07)	0.07 (0.16)	0.04 (0.09)
Difference in state fentanyl seizures per 100 000 population			0.09** (0.03)	0.23** (0.07)	0.24*** (0.05)	0.64*** (0.13)
Difference in jobs per 100 Black workers × difference in state fentanyl seizures per 100 000 population					−0.01*** (<0.01)	−0.56*** (0.14)
Controls						
Difference in county-level percentage of						
Black residents	−4.08** (1.34)	−0.21** (0.07)	−4.24** (1.31)	−0.22** (0.07)	−3.90** (1.27)	−0.20** (0.07)
Male residents	2.48 (6.65)	0.03 (0.07)	1.66 (6.51)	0.02 (0.07)	−0.46 (6.31)	> −0.01 (0.07)
Residents aged ≥ 65 y	−0.17 (2.64)	> −0.01 (0.07)	−0.08 (2.58)	> −0.01 (0.07)	0.17 (2.49)	< 0.01 (0.06)
Residents aged ≥ 25 y without a high-school diploma	−3.53* (1.43)	−0.18* (0.07)	−3.17* (1.40)	−0.17* (0.07)	−3.67** (1.36)	−0.19** (0.07)
Veterans	0.03 (2.89)	< 0.01 (0.07)	0.80 (2.83)	0.02 (0.07)	1.00 (2.74)	0.02 (0.06)
Vacant housing	−0.63 (0.63)	−0.07 (0.07)	−0.54 (0.61)	−0.06 (0.06)	−0.75 (0.59)	−0.08 (0.06)
Difference in county-level						
Unemployment rate, %	0.28 (0.86)	0.02 (0.07)	0.16 (0.84)	0.01 (0.07)	0.39 (0.82)	0.03 (0.07)
Median household income, in $1000 s	0.03 (0.31)	0.01 (0.08)	> −0.01 (0.31)	> −0.01 (0.08)	0.05 (0.30)	0.01 (0.08)
Opioid prescribing rate, per 100 population	−0.31** (0.10)	−0.23** (0.07)	−0.25* (0.10)	−0.19* (0.07)	−0.26** (0.10)	−0.19** (0.07)
Region						
Midwest (Ref)	0	0	0	0	0	0
Northeast	−2.33 (3.86)	−0.05 (0.08)	−4.16 (3.82)	−0.09 (0.08)	−1.62 (3.74)	−0.03 (0.08)
South	−13.86*** (3.61)	−0.35*** (0.09)	−11.62** (3.60)	−0.30** (0.09)	−10.90** (3.48)	−0.28** (0.09)
West	−8.58 (4.60)	−0.15 (0.08)	−4.72 (4.66)	−0.09 (0.08)	−3.60 (4.51)	−0.06 (0.08)
Goodness-of-fit statistics						
Adjusted R^2	0.17		0.21		0.26	
F statistics (*df*1, *df*2)	4.44*** (13, 200)		5.04*** (14, 199)		6.08*** (15, 198)	

Note. The age-adjusted drug overdose mortality rate measures the number of deaths per 100 000 population. Unemployment rate is calculated as the percentage of individuals in the labor force who are unemployed within the county. The differences in the variables were obtained by taking the differences between the value in 2018 to 2021 and the value in 2010 to 2013. The analytic sample consists of 214 counties with at least 10 drug-involved overdose deaths among non-Hispanic Black residents in 2010–2013 and 2018–2021. The fentanyl seizure rates are available only at the state level, and, thus, the moderator does not account for potential intrastate variations. Estimates and standard errors denoted as "< 0.01" or "> –0.01" indicate absolute values smaller than 0.005.
*P < .05; **P < .01; ***P < .001.

DISCUSSION

Our findings offer a salient understanding of the increases in drug mortality rates among Black Americans in the 2010s. First, the drug mortality increases among Black Americans were highest in the Midwest and Northeast counties, especially those with a lower median household income. Economic restructuring (that led to fewer livable-wage jobs in the areas) and increasing presence of heroin and synthetic opioids are considered major drivers of drug mortality in these regions.[4,6]

Second, local employment opportunities were negatively associated with Black Americans' drug mortality, consistent with previous findings that highlighted the role of employment in the US drug epidemic.[7] This suggests that expanding employment opportunities for the Black workforce can be an important component of effective prevention and recovery strategies against substance use risks in the counties with a larger Black community.[8,9]

Lastly, the negative associations between employment opportunities for the Black workforce and drug mortality were stronger in the regions reporting higher increases in state-level fentanyl seizure rates, consistent with fentanyl's role as a moderator of the relationship between job loss and opioid mortality in the general population.[10] That is, in the areas with more active distribution and access to fentanyl, employment opportunities can be more helpful in protecting Black Americans from drug mortality.

PUBLIC HEALTH IMPLICATIONS

Reducing drug mortality among Black Americans may require geographically targeted interventions, focusing on the Midwest and Northeast counties with lower incomes. Such efforts may include improving employment opportunities[11,12] for the Black workforce through job creation and workforce development (including comprehensive skills and training packages for individuals in recovery) to better align Black workforce skills with the demands of the local labor market, especially in the regions with higher increases in fentanyl seizure rates. AJPH

ABOUT THE AUTHORS

Sehun Oh is with the College of Social Work, The Ohio State University, Columbus. Manuel Cano is with the School of Social Work, Arizona State University, Phoenix.

CORRESPONDENCE

Correspondence should be sent to Sehun Oh, 1947 College Rd, Columbus, OH 43210 (e-mail: oh.570@osu.edu). Reprints can be ordered at https://ajph.org by clicking the "Reprints" link.

PUBLICATION INFORMATION

Full Citation: Oh S, Cano M. Black Americans' drug mortality increases and local employment opportunities, 2010–2021. *Am J Public Health*. 2024;114(7):729–732.

Acceptance Date: February 27, 2024.

DOI: https://doi.org/10.2105/AJPH.2024.307646

CONTRIBUTORS

S. Oh led conceptualization, design of methodology, and writing. M. Cano led data curation and statistical analyses and contributed to conceptualization and writing.

ACKNOWLEDGMENTS

Research reported in this article was supported by the National Institute on Drug Abuse of the National Institutes of Health under award number K01DA057514.

Note. The content is solely the responsibility of the authors and does not necessarily represent the official views of the National Institutes of Health.

CONFLICTS OF INTEREST

The authors report no conflicts of interest.

HUMAN PARTICIPANT PROTECTION

This study was determined to be exempt from the institutional review board at Arizona State University (where statistical analyses were conducted) based on 45 CFR 46.102(e1).

REFERENCES

1. Overdose death rates increased significantly for Black, American Indian/Alaska Native people in 2020. Atlanta, GA: Centers for Disease Control and Prevention; 2022.
2. Dasgupta N, Beletsky L, Ciccarone D. Opioid crisis: no easy fix to its social and economic determinants. *Am J Public Health*. 2018;108(2):182–186. https://doi.org/10.2105/AJPH.2017.304187
3. Friedman JR, Hansen H. Evaluation of increases in drug overdose mortality rates in the US by race and ethnicity before and during the COVID-19 pandemic. *JAMA Psychiatry*. 2022;79(4):379–381. https://doi.org/10.1001/jamapsychiatry.2022.0004
4. Monnat SM. The contributions of socioeconomic and opioid supply factors to U.S. drug mortality rates: urban-rural and within-rural differences. *J Rural Stud*. 2019;68:319–335. https://doi.org/10.1016/j.jrurstud.2018.12.004
5. Mars SG, Rosenblum D, Ciccarone D. Illicit fentanyls in the opioid street market: desired or imposed? *Addiction*. 2019;114(5):774–780. https://doi.org/10.1111/add.14474
6. Jalal H, Buchanich JM, Roberts MS, Balmert LC, Zhang K, Burke DS. Changing dynamics of the drug overdose epidemic in the United States from 1979 through 2016. *Science*. 2018;361(6408): eaau1184. https://doi.org/10.1126/science.aau1184
7. Betz MR, Jones LE. Wage and employment growth in America's drug epidemic: is all growth created equal? *Am J Agric Econ*. 2018;100(5): 1357–1374. https://doi.org/10.1093/ajae/aay069
8. Park JN, Rouhani S, Beletsky L, Vincent L, Saloner B, Sherman SG. Situating the continuum of overdose risk in the social determinants of health: a new conceptual framework. *Milbank Q*. 2020;98(3): 700–746. https://doi.org/10.1111/1468-0009.12470
9. Hawk K, Grau LE, Fiellin DA, et al. A qualitative study of emergency department patients who survived an opioid overdose: perspectives on treatment and unmet needs. *Acad Emerg Med*. 2021;28(5):542–552. https://doi.org/10.1111/acem.14197
10. Dean A, Kimmel S. Free trade and opioid overdose death in the United States [erratum in *SSM Popul Health*. 2020;12:100714]. *SSM Popul Health*. 2019;8:100409. https://doi.org/10.1016/j.ssmph.2019.100409
11. Manyika J, Lund S, Chui M, et al. Jobs lost, jobs gained: workforce transitions in a time of automation. McKinsey Global Institute; 2017.
12. Sigurdsson SO, Ring BM, O'Reilly K, Silverman K. Barriers to employment among unemployed drug users: age predicts severity. *Am J Drug Alcohol Abuse*. 2012;38(6):580–587. https://doi.org/10.3109/00952990.2011.643976

Changes in Racial and Ethnic Inequities in Pregnancy-Associated Death in the United States During the COVID-19 Pandemic

Claire E. Margerison, PhD, MPH, Xueshi Wang, MA, Sidra Goldman-Mellor, PhD, MPH, Maria Muzik, MD, MSc, and Alison Gemmill, PhD, MPH

See also Brown and DuBois, p. 666.

Objectives. To examine changes in cause-specific pregnancy-associated deaths during the COVID-19 pandemic by race and ethnicity and assess changes in racial and ethnic inequities in pregnancy-associated deaths.

Methods. We used US vital statistics mortality data from 2018 to 2021 to identify pregnancy-associated deaths among females aged 15 to 44 years. We calculated crude pregnancy-associated death rates (deaths per 100 000 live births) by year, cause, and race/ethnicity, percent change in death rate, and the inequity (difference) in rate for each racial or ethnic group compared with non-Hispanic White people.

Results. The pregnancy-associated death rate for obstetric, drug-related, homicide, and other causes of death increased during 2020, and obstetric deaths continued to increase in 2021. Overall estimates mask 2021 increases in drug-related deaths among Hispanic, non-Hispanic American Indian and Alaska Native (AI/AN), and non-Hispanic Asian people; increases in homicide among most racial and ethnic groups; and increases in suicide among Hispanic, non-Hispanic AI/AN, and non-Hispanic Asian people.

Conclusions. We found disproportionate increases in pregnancy-associated deaths from nonobstetric causes among minoritized racial and ethnic groups during the COVID-19 pandemic. (*Am J Public Health.* 2024;114(7):733–742. https://doi.org/10.2105/AJPH.2024.307651)

AJPH July 2024, Vol. 114, No. 7

Pregnancy-related deaths (i.e., death during pregnancy or within 1 year of the end of pregnancy from causes related to or aggravated by pregnancy[1]) increased during the COVID-19 pandemic, with larger increases in 2021 compared with 2020[2,3] and particularly large increases among American Indian and Alaska Native (AI/AN) people.[2] Furthermore, deaths during pregnancy or the first year postpartum from causes not captured under "pregnancy-related"—including drug-related deaths, homicides, and suicides—make up a large and growing portion of all pregnancy-associated mortality,[4] and these drug-related deaths and homicides increased 55% and 41%, respectively, during the early pandemic.[5,6] Compared with non-Hispanic White pregnant and postpartum people, non-Hispanic Black people experience higher rates of pregnancy-associated death from obstetric causes and homicide, while AI/AN people experience higher rates of pregnancy-associated death from obstetric causes, drugs, homicide, and suicide.[2,4,7]

Racial and ethnic inequities in pregnancy-associated death stem from structurally racist and unjust systems of power, privilege, and resource allocation rooted in our nation's history of genocide, enslavement, segregation, mistreatment, and erasure of Indigenous and Black people as well as other minoritized people.[8] Today, Black, AI/AN, and other minoritized people experience unequal access to high-quality, respectful, and culturally appropriate health care.[9–12] Implicit biases among health care providers—such as beliefs that Black patients experience less pain[13]—and mistreatment of patients of color during pregnancy and childbirth[14] contribute to disparities in maternal health.[15] Structural racism also results in inequities in access to safe and affordable housing, transportation, childcare, education, and employment,[8] all of which directly impact health during pregnancy and postpartum as well as the ability to obtain health care, particularly in an emergency when immediate access to care can prevent death (e.g., postpartum hemorrhage or sepsis, drug overdose, or mental health emergency). Structural racism further defines the environments in which pregnant and postpartum people grew up, live, and work, putting historically oppressed groups at higher risk of exposure to environmental pollution and toxins, violence, and substance use, and constraining choices around diet, physical activity, contraception, and other health behaviors.[8]

Existing inequities in pregnancy-associated death may have been impacted by the COVID-19 pandemic as risk factors associated with pregnancy-associated death—including lack of preventive care access, intimate partner violence, psychosocial stress, unemployment, and financial distress—all increased during the pandemic.[16–18] Moreover, Black, AI/AN, Pacific Islander, and Hispanic communities were disproportionately impacted by COVID-19 morbidity and mortality.[19]

We therefore aimed to expand on previous work demonstrating increases in pregnancy-related mortality during the COVID-19 pandemic by examining changes from 2018 to 2021 in pregnancy-associated deaths from all causes (i.e., obstetric, drug-related, homicide, suicide, and other). We estimated changes in cause-specific pregnancy-associated deaths by race and ethnicity and assessed whether inequities in cause-specific pregnancy-associated deaths narrowed, widened, or stayed the same during the pandemic.

METHODS

We used US vital statistics mortality data (i.e., death certificate records) from 2018, 2019, 2020, and 2021 to identify pregnancy-associated deaths among female decedents aged 15 to 44 years who were US residents.[20] We obtained the count of live births from the Centers for Disease Control and Prevention WONDER database, also for US residents aged 15 to 44 years. We limited our analysis to deaths and births occurring between April and December of 2018, 2019, 2020, and 2021 to correspond to the months of the COVID-19 pandemic in 2020.

Measures

We first identified deaths as pregnancy-associated if the pregnancy checkbox on the death certificate indicated the decedent was pregnant at the time of death, not pregnant but pregnant within 42 days of death, or not pregnant but pregnant 43 days to 1 year before death. Second, we used *International Classification of Diseases, 10th Revision* (*ICD-10*; Geneva, Switzerland: World Health Organization; 1992) codes to identify additional deaths from causes related to pregnancy, childbirth, and the puerperium (*ICD-10* codes O00–O96, O98, O99), or obstetrical tetanus (A34) not noted with the checkbox. Finally, we classified pregnancy-associated deaths based on underlying cause of death *ICD-10* codes into the following categories: obstetric causes, drug-related causes (unintentional or of undetermined intent), suicide, homicide, and all other causes (all causes that did not fall into one of the previous categories; see Table A, available as a supplement to the online version of this article at https://ajph.org, for *ICD-10* codes.)

Race and ethnicity were assigned based on the death certificate and categorized following the Office of Management and Budget classifications. Decedents listed as Hispanic were categorized as Hispanic, and non-Hispanic decedents were categorized based on their indicated race as White, Black, AI/AN, Asian, Native Hawaiian and other Pacific Islander (NH/PI), or multiple races.

We calculated the crude pregnancy-associated death rate

$$(1)\quad \left(\frac{\#\ pregnancy-associated\ deaths}{\#\ live\ births}\right) \times 100\,000$$

for April to December of each year for each cause of death and for each racial and ethnic group and generated 95% confidence intervals (CIs) for those rates assuming a χ^2 distribution. We note that our measure is also commonly referred to as the pregnancy-associated death ratio as the denominator does not equal the population at risk.

Small Cell Sizes

In some years and for some causes of death, estimates for the non-Hispanic Asian, non-Hispanic AI/AN, non-Hispanic NH/PI, and non-Hispanic multiple race categories were based on fewer than 10 deaths. We clearly note in all tables and figures where estimates are based on fewer than 10 deaths, but we chose not to suppress or exclude these estimates because reporting mortality for all racial and ethnic groups is the first step to recognizing and preventing specific causes of death in all groups.[21,22] To increase cell sizes, we also combined years of data for the least common causes of death (i.e., homicide, suicide, and other causes), grouping 2018 and 2019 as before the COVID-19 pandemic and 2020 and 2021 as during the pandemic.

Percent Change Over Time

For all groups and causes of death, we calculated the percent change in pregnancy-associated death rate across years or from before to during the pandemic using the incidence rate (IR) command in StataMP version 16 (StataCorp LP, College Station, TX) to obtain rate ratios (which can be transformed to percentage by subtracting 1 and multiplying by 100) and 95% CIs.

Inequity Measure

We then calculated the ratio difference and associated 95% CI by subtracting the cause-specific pregnancy-associated death ratio for each racial and ethnic group from the ratio for non-Hispanic White people. We chose non-Hispanic Whites as the reference group because this group has historically experienced the least oppression, systemic bias, and structural racism. A health inequity arises when a group that is already systemically disadvantaged is at a further disadvantage in terms of health.[23] Thus, ratio differences greater than zero (indicating that the racial or ethnic group in question had a higher pregnancy-associated death ratio compared with non-Hispanic White people) indicate a health inequity. We assessed whether ratio differences and health inequities in cause-specific pregnancy-associated death rate increased, decreased, or stayed the same across the study period.

RESULTS

We identified a total of 6666 pregnancy-associated deaths from 2018 to 2021 (deaths in April through December only). Compared with people with a live birth during the study period, those with pregnancy-associated deaths were more frequently aged 35 to 44 years, non-Hispanic Black or non-Hispanic AI/AN, not married, and with less than a college education (Table B, available as a supplement to the online version of this article at https://ajph.org). Of these deaths during pregnancy and postpartum, 57.6% were from obstetric causes, 17.7% were drug-related, 7.4% were homicides, 4.9% were suicides, and 12.3% were from other causes, primarily motor vehicle accidents. Overall pregnancy-associated deaths increased 9.4% from 2018 to 2019, 35.0% from 2019 to 2020, and 13.7% from 2020 to 2021 (Table C, available as a supplement to the online version of this article at https://ajph.org). In the first year of the COVID-19 pandemic (from 2019 to 2020) almost all causes of death (except for suicide) increased, with obstetric deaths increasing by 28.4%, drug-related deaths by 55.3%, homicide by 41.2%, and other causes by 56.7% (Table C). From 2020 to 2021, however, obstetric deaths increased another 30.5%, while changes to other causes of death were not statistically significant (Table C).

Racial/Ethnic Disparities

Across the 4-year study period, non-Hispanic Black, non-Hispanic AI/AN, and non-Hispanic NH/PI people had the highest death rate from obstetric causes (Figure 1). Non-Hispanic AI/AN people had the highest pregnancy-associated death rate from drug-related causes (Figure 2), suicide (Table D3, available as a supplement to the online version of this article at https://ajph.org), and other causes (Table D1, available as a supplement to the online version of this article at https://ajph.org); non-Hispanic Black people had the highest pregnancy-associated death ratio from homicide (Table D2, available as a supplement to the online version of this article at https://ajph.org).

Changes Over Time by Race and Ethnicity

Obstetric deaths. Pregnancy and postpartum deaths from obstetric causes increased among almost all racial/ethnic groups from 2019 to 2020 and from 2020 to 2021 (Figure 1). Non-Hispanic AI/AN people experienced a substantial and statistically significant ($P < .05$) increase of 110% in obstetric deaths from 2020 to 2021 (Figure 1). The obstetric death ratio for non-Hispanic Black pregnant and postpartum people also increased significantly across the study period, from 53.1 deaths per 100 000 live births in 2018 to 101.7 per 100 000 in 2021 (Figure 1). Although the obstetric death rates among Hispanic and non-Hispanic Asian people were relatively low compared with other groups in 2018, both groups experienced increases in obstetric deaths during the pandemic, with statistically significant increases of 49.1 and 35.4 among Hispanic people from 2019 to 2020 and 2020 to 2021, respectively (Figure 1).

Figure 2 shows the ratio difference in the pregnancy-associated death ratio from obstetric causes among each racial and ethnic group relative to non-Hispanic White people. Values above zero indicate an inequity (i.e., in that year, the racial or ethnic group had

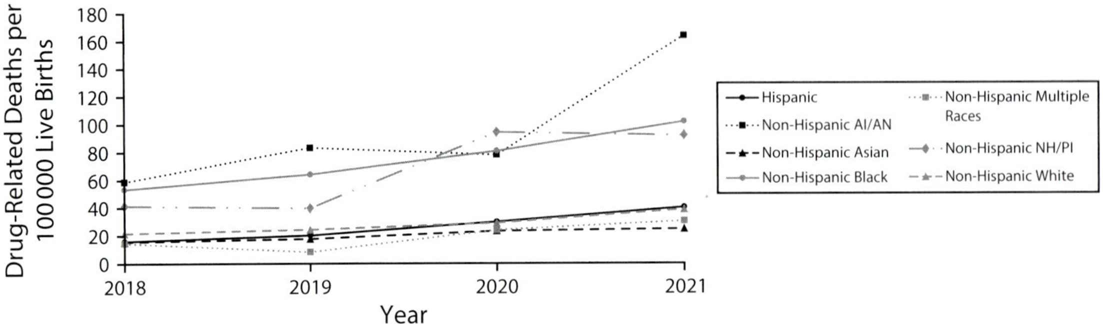

	2018	2019	2020	2021	Percent Change in PAD Rate		
	PAD Rate (95% CI)	PAD Rate (95% CI)	PAD Rate (95% CI)	PAD Rate (95% CI)	2018–2019	2019–2020	2020–2021
Hispanic	15.5 (12.7, 18.8)	19.7 (16.5, 23.4)	29.4 (25.4, 33.9)	39.8 (35.2, 44.8)	27.3	49.1*	35.4*
Non-Hispanic White	21.2 (18.9, 23.7)	23.8 (21.4, 26.5)	28.6 (25.8, 31.5)	38.3 (35.2, 41.6)	12.1	19.8*	34.2*
Non-Hispanic Black	53.1 (46.4, 60.6)	63.9 (56.5, 72.1)	80.7 (72.2, 90.0)	101.7 (92.0, 112.1)	20.3*	26.3*	26.0*
Non-Hispanic AI/AN	58.5 (31.2, 100.1)	83.1 (49.3, 131.4)	77.9 (44.5, 126.5)	163.8 (112.7, 230.0)	42	-6.3	110.2*
Non-Hispanic Asian	15.1 (10.0, 21.8)	17.3 (11.8, 24.4)	22.8 (16.1, 31.3)	24.2 (17.4, 32.9)	14.2	32.1	6.4
Non-Hispanic NH/PI[a]	40.9 (8.4, 119.7)	39.3 (8.1, 115.0)	94.2 (37.9, 194.1)	91.8 (36.9, 189.1)	-3.9	133.3	-2.6
Non-Hispanic Multiple Races[a]	14.1 (6.4, 26.7)	7.8 (2.5, 18.1)	23.4 (13.1, 38.6)	29.9 (18.3, 46.2)	-44.9	201.4*	27.9
Total	24.3 (22.5, 26.2)	28.4 (26.5, 30.5)	36.5 (34.3, 38.9)	47.7 (45.1, 50.3)	17.1*	28.4*	30.5*

FIGURE 1— Obstetric Pregnancy-Associated Death Rates and Percent Change by Race and Ethnicity: US Vital Statistics Data, April to December, 2018–2021

Note. AI/AN = American Indian and Alaska Native; CI = confidence interval; NH/PI = Native Hawaiian and other Pacific Islander; PAD = pregnancy-associated death. Death rate indicates number of deaths per 100 000 live births.
[a]Obstetric pregnancy-associated death rates for non-Hispanic NH/PI and non-Hispanic multiple race rely on fewer than 10 deaths in some years.
*Percent change statistically significantly different from zero at $P < .05$.

more pregnancy-associated deaths per 100 000 live births from that cause relative to non-Hispanic White people). Hispanic pregnant and postpartum people had lower obstetric death rates than non-Hispanic White people in 2018, but during 2020 and 2021 there was no significant difference between non-Hispanic White and Hispanic people. Substantial inequities in obstetric deaths existed for non-Hispanic Black, non-Hispanic AI/AN, and non-Hispanic NH/PI people compared with non-Hispanic White people before the pandemic, and those inequities widened during 2020 and 2021 (Figure 2).

Drug-related deaths. Patterns of drug-related pregnancy-associated death during the pandemic differed among racial and ethnic groups (Figure 3). Drug-related deaths among non-Hispanic Black pregnant and postpartum people increased before and during the early pandemic period (significant increases of 165.8% from 2018 to 2019 and 78.2% from 2019 to 2020) but not from 2020 to 2021 (Figure 3). Drug-related pregnancy-associated deaths increased from 2019 to 2020 among Hispanic, non-Hispanic White, and non-Hispanic AI/AN people and those reporting multiple races (59.1%, 49.2%, 35.6%, and 166.0%, respectively), and continued to increase among Hispanic and non-Hispanic AI/AN people from 2020 to 2021 (57.1% and 58.6%, respectively; Figure 3), but none of those increases reached statistical significance.

The inequity in drug-related deaths among non-Hispanic AI/AN people

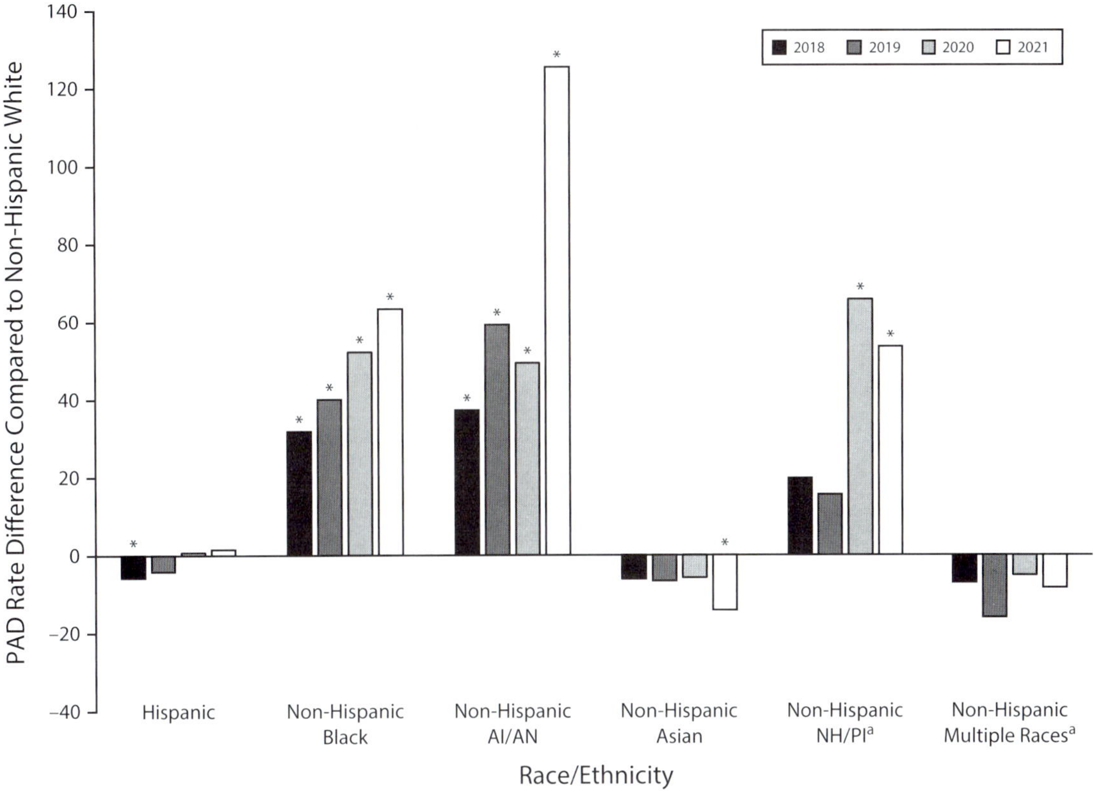

	PAD Rate Difference (95% CI)					
	Hispanic	Non-Hispanic Black	Non-Hispanic AI/AN	Non-Hispanic Asian	Non-Hispanic NH/PI[a]	Non-Hispanic Multiple Races[a]
2018	−5.7 (−9.7, −1.7)	31.9 (26.2, 37.7)	37.3 (17.8, 56.9)	−6.1 (−13.0, 0.8)	19.7 (−13.8, 53.2)	−7.2 (−18.6, 4.3)
2019	−4.1 (−8.5, 0.2)	40.1 (33.9, 46.3)	59.3 (38.2, 80.4)	−6.6 (−13.9, 50.3)	15.5 (−19.3, 50.3)	−16.2 (−28.1, −4.1)
2020	0.8 (−4.2, 5.8)	52.2 (45.1, 59.2)	49.4 (25.8, 72.9)	−5.8 (−14.3, 2.7)	65.7 (26.9, 101.4)	−5.2 (−18.5, 8.2)
2021	1.5 (−4.2, 7.1)	63.4 (55.4, 71.4)	125.4 (97.6, 153.3)	−14.1 (−23.7, −4.4)	53.5 (9.3, 97.7)	−8.4 (−23.5, 6.7)

FIGURE 2— Difference in Pregnancy-Associated Death Rate From Obstetric Causes Among Each Racial and Ethnic Group Relative to Non-Hispanic White People: US Vital Statistics Data, April to December, 2018–2021

Note. AI/AN = American Indian and Alaska Native; CI = confidence interval; NH/PI = Native Hawaiian and other Pacific Islander; PAD = pregnancy-associated death. Cause-specific pregnancy-associated death rate for each racial and ethnic group were subtracted from non-Hispanic White. Values > 0 indicate an inequity, or that the racial or ethnic group had more pregnancy-associated deaths from this cause relative to non-Hispanic White people.
[a]At least 1 data point is based on < 10 deaths.
* Pregnancy-associated death ratio in this group and year is statistically significantly different from non-Hispanic White ratio in this year at $P < .05$.

compared with non-Hispanic White people grew steadily before and during the pandemic (Figure 4). In 2018, the drug-related death ratio for non-Hispanic AI/AN pregnant and postpartum people was not statistically significantly different from the ratio for non-Hispanic White people, but in 2021, it was 52.2 deaths per 100 000 live births higher (Figure 4). Most other racial and ethnic groups had consistently lower pregnancy-associated death rates from drugs compared with non-Hispanic White people (Figure 4).

Homicide. All groups except for non-Hispanic multiple races experienced increases of 40% or more in pregnancy-associated homicide during the pandemic period, with statistically significant increases among non-Hispanic White and non-Hispanic Black people

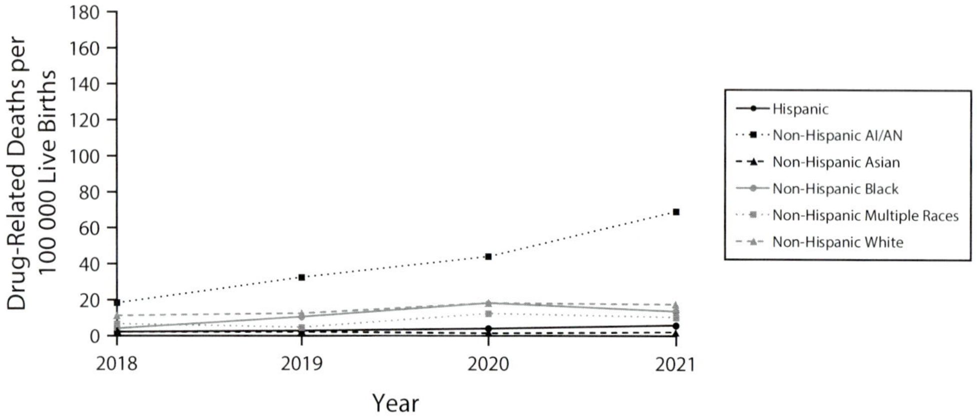

	2018	2019	2020	2021	Percent Change in PAD Rate		
	PAD Rate (95% CI)	PAD Rate (95% CI)	PAD Rate (95% CI)	PAD Rate (95% CI)	2018–2019	2019–2020	2020–2021
Hispanic	2.1 (1.1, 3.5)	2.2 (1.2, 3.7)	3.5 (2.2, 5.3)	5.5 (3.9, 7.6)	6.7	58.3	57.4
Non-Hispanic White	10.9 (9.3, 12.7)	12 (10.3, 13.9)	17.9 (15.7, 20.2)	17.2 (15.2, 19.5)	9.3	49.5*	-3.5
Non-Hispanic Black	3.8 (2.2, 6.2)	10.1 (7.3, 13.6)	18.0 (14.1, 22.7)	13.3 (10.0, 17.4)	162.5*	79.0*	−26.4
Non-Hispanic AI/AN[a]	18.0 (4.9, 46.1)	32.3 (13.0, 66.6)	43.8 (20.0, 83.2)	69.5 (38.0, 116.6)	79.5	35.6	58.5
Non-Hispanic Asian[a]	1.6 (0.3, 4.7)	1.6 (0.3, 4.7)	1.2 (0.2, 4.3)	1.8 (0.4, 5.2)	0.1	−25.9	47.9
Non-Hispanic Multiple Races[a]	6.3 (1.7, 16.0)	4.7 (1.0, 13.6)	12.5 (5.39, 24.6)	10.5 (4.2, 21.6)	−25.6	167.9	−16.0
Total	7.1 (6.2, 8.2)	8.7 (7.6, 9.8)	13.4 (12.1, 14.9)	13.1 (11.8, 14.5)	21.0*	55.3*	-2.9

FIGURE 3— Drug-Related Pregnancy-Associated Death Rates and Percent Change by Race and Ethnicity: US Vital Statistics Data, April to December, 2018–2021

Note. AI/AN = American Indian and Alaska Native; CI = confidence interval; PAD = pregnancy-associated death. Pregnancy-associated death rate indicates the number of deaths per 100 000 live births. Non-Hispanic Native Hawaiian and other Pacific Islander people are not included because this group had no drug-related deaths in multiple years.

[a]Drug-related pregnancy-associated death rates for non-Hispanic AI/AN, non-Hispanic Asian, and non-Hispanic multiple race rely on fewer than 10 deaths in some years.

*Percent change statistically significantly different from zero at $P<.05$.

(Figure A1 and Table D1, available as supplements to the online version of this article at https://ajph.org). Non-Hispanic Black pregnant and postpartum people had the highest homicide death ratio in the prepandemic period at 12.2 per 100 000 live births, and this ratio increased by 73.4% during the pandemic to 21.2 per 100 000 (Table D1).

Inequities in pregnancy-associated death rate from homicide existed for Hispanic, non-Hispanic Black, and non-Hispanic multiple race groups relative to non-Hispanic White people both before and during the pandemic (Figure B1 and Table E1, available as supplements to the online version of this article at https://ajph.org). The inequity in homicide deaths for non-Hispanic AI/AN people compared with non-Hispanic White people was not statistically significantly different from zero before the pandemic but increased to a statistically significant 5 additional deaths per 100 000 live births during the pandemic (Figure B1 and Supplemental Table E1).

Suicide. Non-Hispanic White and non-Hispanic Black pregnant and postpartum people experienced declines in pregnancy-associated suicide during the pandemic, but most other groups experienced increases. That is, suicide increased 23.4% among Hispanic people, 7.8% among non-Hispanic AI/AN people,

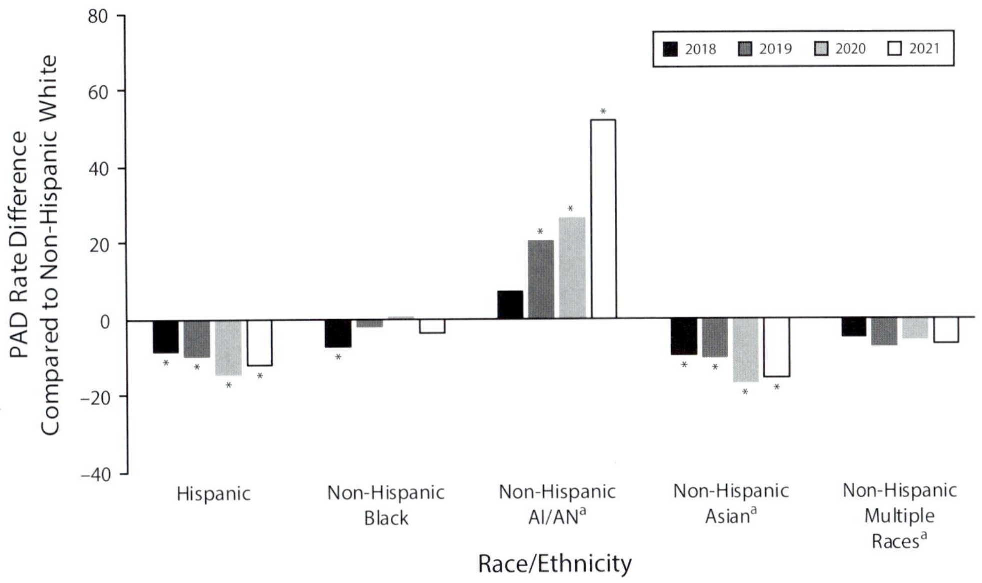

	PAD Rate Difference (95% CI)				
	Hispanic	Non-Hispanic Black	Non-Hispanic AI/AN[a]	Non-Hispanic Asian[a]	Non-Hispanic Multiple Races[a]
2018	−8.6 (−11.5, −6.2)	−7.1 (−10.4, −3.8)	7.1 (−6.8, 21.0)	−9.3 (−14.1, −4.5)	−4.7 (−12.9, 3.5)
2019	−9.7 (−12.5, −7.0)	−1.9 (−5.6, 1.8)	20.4 (5.5, 35.2)	−10.3 (−15.4, −5.3)	−7.2 (−15.8, 1.2)
2020	−14.4 (−17.7, −11.0)	0.1 (−4.6, 4.8)	26.0 (7.3, 44.6)	−16.7 (−23.1, −10.2)	−5.4 (−15.9, 5.1)
2021	−11.7 (−15.0, −8.4)	−3.9 (−8.4, 0.6)	52.2 (33.6, 70.9)	−15.5 (−21.8, −9.2)	−6.8 (−16.9, 3.3)

FIGURE 4— Difference in Pregnancy-Associated Death Rate From Drug-Related Causes Among Each Racial and Ethnic Group Relative to Non-Hispanic White People: US Vital Statistics Data, April to December, 2018–2021

Note. AI/AN = American Indian and Alaska Native; CI = confidence interval; PAD = pregnancy-associated death. Cause-specific pregnancy-associated death rate for each racial and ethnic group subtracted from non-Hispanic White. Values > 0 indicate an inequity, or that the racial or ethnic group had more pregnancy-associated deaths from this cause relative to non-Hispanic White people. Non-Hispanic Native Hawaiian and other Pacific Islander people are not included because this group had no drug-related deaths in multiple years.
[a]At least 1 data point is based on < 10 deaths.
*Pregnancy-associated death ratio in this group and year is statistically significantly different from non-Hispanic White ratio in this year at $P < .05$.

65.6% among non-Hispanic Asian people, and 30.7% among non-Hispanic people reporting multiple races (Figure A2 and Table D2, available as supplements to the online version of this article at https://ajph.org); none of these percent changes were statistically significantly different from zero.

Before the pandemic, a nonstatistically significant inequity in pregnancy-associated suicide existed for non-Hispanic AI/AN people, who experienced 5.1 more suicides per 100 000 live births compared with non-Hispanic White people in 2018 and 2019, and this inequity increased to a statistically significant 6.4 more suicides per 100 000 live births compared with non-Hispanic White people in 2020 and 2021 (Figure B2 and Table E2, available as supplements to the online version of this article at https://ajph.org). For most other racial and ethnic groups, the pregnancy-associated death ratio difference for suicide became closer to zero during the pandemic, indicating that the relative advantage in terms of pregnancy-associated suicide narrowed for these groups, compared with non-Hispanic White people (Figure B2 and Table E2).

Other causes of death. Pregnancy-associated deaths from all other causes combined increased among all racial and ethnic groups except for non-Hispanic multiple race people during

AJPH July 2024, Vol. 114, No. 7

the pandemic (Figure A3 and Table D3, available as supplements to the online version of this article at https://ajph.org). Non-Hispanic AI/AN people and non-Hispanic Black people had the highest pregnancy-associated death rate from other causes overall, and both groups experienced increases during the pandemic (41.0% and 29.0%, respectively); none of these percent changes were statistically significantly different from zero. Inequities in deaths from other causes also exist between non-Hispanic AI/AN and non-Hispanic Black people and non-Hispanic White people, and those inequities increased during the pandemic (Figure B3 and Table E3, available as supplements to the online version of this article at https://ajph.org). The inequity for non-Hispanic AI/AN relative to non-Hispanic White people increased substantially from 17.2 (95% CI = 6.8, 27.7) more deaths per 100 000 live births in 2019 to 39.7 (95% CI = 26.1, 53.2) in 2020.

DISCUSSION

Our analysis of nationwide birth and death records from 2018 to 2021 found that, in the first year of the COVID-19 pandemic (from 2019 to 2020), pregnancy-associated deaths from all causes except for suicide (i.e., obstetric causes, drug-related causes, homicide, and all other causes combined) increased between 30% and 60%. In 2021, however, obstetric deaths increased another 31%, but other causes of death did not significantly change. These overall figures mask disproportionate increases in cause-specific pregnancy-associated death among minoritized racial and ethnic groups. Not only did many racial and ethnic groups experience an overall increase in pregnancy-associated deaths from obstetric causes during the pandemic, but also the inequity in obstetric death compared with non-Hispanic White people increased for Hispanic, non-Hispanic Black, non-Hispanic AI/AN, and non-Hispanic NH/PI people. While drug-related pregnancy-associated death rates increased for many groups from 2019 to 2020, non-Hispanic AI/AN people experienced a substantial inequity in drug-related deaths compared with non-Hispanic White people that increased consistently across the study period. Pregnancy-associated homicide increased for almost all racial and ethnic groups during the pandemic, and the inequity in homicide increased for Hispanic, non-Hispanic Black, and non-Hispanic AI/AN people compared with non-Hispanic White people. Although pregnancy-associated suicide appeared to decline overall during the pandemic, Hispanic, non-Hispanic AI/AN, non-Hispanic Asian, and non-Hispanic multiple race people all experienced increases in suicide (though not statistically significant).

Our study includes estimates of pregnancy-associated death by cause for some racial and ethnic groups with small numbers of deaths. While we acknowledge that these small cell sizes do place limits on statistical testing and interpretation, suppression and exclusion of data for racial and ethnic groups because of small numbers is a noted public health problem labeled by scholars as data genocide.[21,22] We believe publishing these pregnancy-associated death estimates for the smaller racial and ethnic groups reflects a public health justice approach crucial to driving awareness and policy change. Indeed, our analysis shows substantial inequities in pregnancy-associated death among non-Hispanic AI/AN people for almost all causes of death, highlighting the urgent need for increased attention and resources from the public health community to address the unique health challenges faced by these groups as the result of centuries of settler colonialism, genocide, and erasure. Our findings also illuminate pandemic-related increases in pregnancy-associated death (i.e., obstetric causes, drug-related deaths, homicide, suicide, and other causes) among Hispanic and non-Hispanic Asian pregnant and postpartum people, groups often assumed to be "resilient" or to have "paradoxically" low rates of adverse outcomes. Finally, we provide estimates for non-Hispanic NH/PI and non-Hispanic people reporting multiple races. While numbers of both live births and deaths in these groups are small and must be interpreted with caution, our findings suggest these 2 groups represent important populations with potential inequities in pregnancy-associated mortality deserving of further monitoring and research.

Patterns in pregnancy-associated death mirrored those seen for the same causes of death in the general population. Among women of reproductive age in general, non-Hispanic AI/AN women had the highest all-cause mortality rates over the past 2 decades.[24] Moreover, suicide rates among White females overall declined 3% between 2019 and 2021 but increased among females of other racial/ethnic groups, resulting in a closing of racial/ethnic gaps similar to those described in our data (https://www.cdc.gov/injury/wisqars). Our findings also somewhat parallel trends in drug overdose in the general population, as drug overdoses accelerated during 2020 and 2021 among both males and females and disproportionately affected non-Hispanic AI/AN and non-Hispanic Black people (for whom mortality increased by 95% and 79% from 2019 to 2021, respectively).[25,26]

Limitations

Important limitations include that substantial misclassification occurs for both pregnancy-associated death and cause of death with death certificate data. The pregnancy checkbox undercounts nonobstetric and late postpartum pregnancy-associated deaths[27] but overcounts obstetric deaths by up to 50%.[28,29] We limited our analysis to decedents younger than 45 years, as errors are more common among older people.[28] Previous reports have also found that approximately half of accidental deaths during pregnancy or postpartum were subsequently identified as probable suicides,[30] meaning that suicide may be undercounted. Underestimation and misclassification of overdose mortality, especially for deaths involving certain types of opioids, also frequently occur.[31,32]

Race and ethnicity are social constructs that change over time and are not easily measured using vital statistics data. People identifying as members of a federally recognized AI/AN nation or tribe may also identify with other race or ethnic groups; when we prioritized AI/AN by putting any death into that category regardless of other race or ethnic group identified,[33] we found an equal number of deaths. Moreover, the AI/AN group does not encompass all Indigenous people living in the United States. We also prioritized Hispanic ethnicity, so people identifying as both Hispanic and Black, Asian, or any other race would be categorized as Hispanic. This may contribute to erasure or undercounting of people identifying with both a minoritized racial group and Hispanic. As self-report of multiple races has increased over time, we cannot determine whether increases in deaths among this group result from changes in risk within the group or changes in the composition of the group. Classifications of racial and ethnic categories on death certificates and birth certificates may also differ for some pregnant and postpartum decedents, although we have no way of measuring this.

Finally, our study would benefit from data from before 2018 with which to establish prepandemic trends in pregnancy-associated death. However, changes to the classification of race and ethnicity, along with states adopting the pregnancy checkbox at different times, prevented us from including data from before 2018 in this study. Despite these data limitations, these are the only data available to examine pregnancy-associated death across all US states.

Public Health Implications

While considerable attention has been paid to the obstetric effects of the pandemic—including elevated risks of maternal mortality and morbidity from COVID-19 infection—our findings highlight that surveillance of all causes of death among pregnant and postpartum individuals within and between racial and ethnic groups remains an important research priority. Here, we show that minoritized racial and ethnic groups bore a disproportionate burden of pregnancy-associated deaths from drug use, homicide, and suicide. Our findings highlight the need for approaches and interventions to address substance use, mental health, and intimate partner violence that center pregnant and postpartum people's lived experience beyond childbirth and that work to dismantle structural barriers, particularly those established by structural racism and settler colonialism. Such approaches may include reconsideration of punitive policies for pregnant and postpartum people who use substances[34]; clinical and policy efforts to address major gaps in screening, education, and treatment about perinatal mental health[35]; and specific interventions to address gaps in social determinants of health such as housing, transportation, childcare, and financial security for pregnant and postpartum people. AJPH

ABOUT THE AUTHORS

Claire E. Margerison is with the Department of Epidemiology and Biostatistics, College of Human Medicine, Michigan State University, East Lansing. Xueshi Wang is with the Department of Economics, College of Social Science, Michigan State University. Sidra Goldman-Mellor is with the Department of Public Health, School of Social Sciences, Humanities, and Arts, University of California, Merced. Maria Muzik is with the Departments of Psychiatry and Obstetrics & Gynecology, University of Michigan–Michigan Medicine, Ann Arbor. Alison Gemmill is with the Department of Population, Family, and Reproductive Health, Johns Hopkins Bloomberg School of Public Health, Baltimore, MD.

CORRESPONDENCE

Correspondence should be sent to Claire E. Margerison, 909 Wilson Rd, Rm 601B, East Lansing, MI 48824 (e-mail: margeris@msu.edu). Reprints can be ordered at https://ajph.org by clicking the "Reprints" link.

PUBLICATION INFORMATION

Full Citation: Margerison CE, Wang X, Goldman-Mellor S, Muzik M, Gemmill A. Changes in racial and ethnic inequities in pregnancy-associated death in the United States during the COVID-19 pandemic. *Am J Public Health*. 2024;114(7): 733–742.

Acceptance Date: March 4, 2024.

DOI: https://doi.org/10.2105/AJPH.2024.307651

CONTRIBUTORS

C. E. Margerison designed the study, obtained data permissions, oversaw the analysis, and drafted and edited the article. X. Wang conducted the data analysis. S. Goldman-Mellor and A. Gemmill contributed to study design, analytic approach, interpretation and presentation of results, and drafting and editing the article. M. Muzik contributed to interpretation of results and drafting and editing the article.

ACKNOWLEDGMENTS

This study was funded by the Eunice Kennedy Shriver National Institute of Child Health and Human Development through R01HD102319 and R01HD102319-02S1 (MPIs: C. E. Margerison and S. Goldman-Mellor).

CONFLICTS OF INTEREST

The authors have no conflicts of interest to declare.

HUMAN PARTICIPANT PROTECTION

This research received institutional review board approval from Michigan State University.

REFERENCES

1. Centers for Disease Control and Prevention. Pregnancy Mortality Surveillance System. November 25, 2020. Available at: https://www.cdc.gov/reproductivehealth/maternal-mortality/pregnancy-mortality-surveillance-system.htm. Accessed December 4, 2020.
2. Thoma ME, Declercq ER. Changes in pregnancy-related mortality associated with the coronavirus disease 2019 (COVID-19) pandemic in the United States. *Obstet Gynecol*. 2023;141(5):911–917. https://doi.org/10.1097/AOG.0000000000005182
3. Hoyert D. Maternal mortality rates in the United States, 2021. Hyattsville, MD: National Center for Health Statistics; 2023. https://doi.org/10.15620/cdc:124678
4. Margerison CE, Roberts MH, Gemmill A, Goldman-Mellor S. Pregnancy-associated deaths due to drugs, suicide, and homicide in the United States, 2010–2019. *Obstet Gynecol*. 2022;139(2):172–180. https://doi.org/10.1097/AOG.0000000000004649
5. Wallace ME. Trends in pregnancy-associated homicide, United States, 2020. *Am J Public Health*. 2022;112(9):1333–1336. https://doi.org/10.2105/AJPH.2022.306937
6. Margerison CE, Wang X, Gemmill A, Goldman-Mellor S. Changes in pregnancy-associated deaths in the US during the COVID-19 pandemic in 2020. *JAMA Netw Open*. 2023;6(2):e2254287. https://doi.org/10.1001/jamanetworkopen.2022.54287
7. Wallace ME, Hoyert D, Williams C, Mendola P. Pregnancy-associated homicide and suicide in 37 US states with enhanced pregnancy surveillance. *Am J Obstet Gynecol*. 2016;215(3):364.e1–364.e10. https://doi.org/10.1016/j.ajog.2016.03.040
8. Hailu EM, Maddali SR, Snowden JM, Carmichael SL, Mujahid MS. Structural racism and adverse maternal health outcomes: a systematic review. *Health Place*. 2022;78:102923. https://doi.org/10.1016/j.healthplace.2022.102923
9. Heck JL, Jones EJ, Bohn D, et al. Maternal mortality among American Indian/Alaska Native women: a scoping review. *J Womens Health (Larchmt)*. 2021;30(2):220–229. https://doi.org/10.1089/jwh.2020.8890
10. Crear-Perry J, Correa-de-Araujo R, Lewis Johnson T, McLemore MR, Neilson E, Wallace M. Social and structural determinants of health inequities in maternal health. *J Womens Health (Larchmt)*. 2021;30(2):230–235. https://doi.org/10.1089/jwh.2020.8882
11. Kozhimannil KB, Interrante JD, Tofte AN, Admon LK. Severe maternal morbidity and mortality among Indigenous women in the United States. *Obstet Gynecol*. 2020;135(2):294–300. https://doi.org/10.1097/AOG.0000000000003647
12. Howell EA. Reducing disparities in severe maternal morbidity and mortality. *Clin Obstet Gynecol*. 2018;61(2):387–399. https://doi.org/10.1097/GRF.0000000000000349
13. Jones SCT, Anderson RE, Gaskin-Wasson AL, Sawyer BA, Applewhite K, Metzger IW. From "crib to coffin": navigating coping from racism-related stress throughout the lifespan of Black Americans. *Am J Orthopsychiatry*. 2020;90(2):267–282. https://doi.org/10.1037/ort0000430
14. Vedam S, Stoll K, Taiwo TK, et al. The Giving Voice to Mothers study: inequity and mistreatment during pregnancy and childbirth in the United States. *Reprod Health*. 2019;16(1):77. https://doi.org/10.1186/s12978-019-0729-2
15. Saluja B, Bryant Z. How implicit bias contributes to racial disparities in maternal morbidity and mortality in the United States. *J Womens Health (Larchmt)*. 2021;30(2):270–273. https://doi.org/10.1089/jwh.2020.8874
16. Piquero AR, Jennings WG, Jemison E, Kaukinen C, Knaul FM. Domestic violence during the COVID-19 pandemic—evidence from a systematic review and meta-analysis. *J Crim Justice*. 2021;74:101806. https://doi.org/10.1016/j.jcrimjus.2021.101806
17. McGinty EE, Presskreischer R, Han H, Barry CL. Psychological distress and loneliness reported by US adults in 2018 and April 2020. *JAMA*. 2020;324(1):93–94. https://doi.org/10.1001/jama.2020.9740
18. Wright A, Salazar A, Mirica M, Volk LA, Schiff GD. The invisible epidemic: neglected chronic disease management during COVID-19. *J Gen Intern Med*. 2020;35(9):2816–2817. https://doi.org/10.1007/s11606-020-06025-4
19. Gawthrop E. Color of coronavirus: COVID-19 deaths analyzed by race and ethnicity. APM Research Lab. Available at: https://www.apmresearchlab.org/covid/deaths-by-race. Accessed June 1, 2023.
20. National Center for Health Statistics. Compressed Mortality File. February 28, 2022. Available at: https://www.cdc.gov/nchs/data_access/cmf.htm. Accessed June 1, 2023.
21. Mays VM, Echo-Hawk A, Cochran SD, Akee R. Data equity in American Indian/Alaska Native populations: respecting sovereign nations' right to meaningful and usable COVID-19 data. *Am J Public Health*. 2022;112(10):1416–1420. https://doi.org/10.2105/AJPH.2022.307043
22. Denetclaw P. Data genocide, maternal mortality, and a return to tradition. *Native News Online*. May 13, 2022. Available at: https://nativenewsonline.net/health/data-genocide-maternal-mortality-and-a-return-to-tradition. Accessed September 27, 2023.
23. Braveman P, Gruskin S. Defining equity in health. *J Epidemiol Community Health*. 2003;57(4):254–258. https://doi.org/10.1136/jech.57.4.254
24. Gemmill A, Berger BO, Crane MA, Margerison CE. Mortality rates among US women of reproductive age, 1999–2019. *Am J Prev Med*. 2022;62(4):548–557. https://doi.org/10.1016/j.amepre.2021.10.009
25. Spencer MR, Miniño AM, Warner M. Drug overdose deaths in the United States, 2001–2021. *NCHS Data Brief*. 2022;(457):1–8. https://doi.org/10.15620/cdc:122556
26. Friedman JR, Hansen H. Evaluation of increases in drug overdose mortality rates in the US by race and ethnicity before and during the COVID-19 pandemic. *JAMA Psychiatry*. 2022;79(4):379–381. https://doi.org/10.1001/jamapsychiatry.2022.0004
27. Horon IL, Cheng D. Effectiveness of pregnancy check boxes on death certificates in identifying pregnancy-associated mortality. *Public Health Rep*. 2011;126(2):195–200. https://doi.org/10.1177/003335491112600210
28. Baeva S, Saxton DL, Ruggiero K, et al. Identifying maternal deaths in Texas using an enhanced method, 2012. *Obstet Gynecol*. 2018;131(5):762–769. https://doi.org/10.1097/AOG.0000000000002565
29. Catalano A, Davis NL, Petersen EE, et al. Pregnant? Validity of the pregnancy checkbox on death certificates in four states, and characteristics associated with pregnancy checkbox errors. *Am J Obstet Gynecol*. 2020;222(3):269.e1–269.e8. https://doi.org/10.1016/j.ajog.2019.10.005
30. California Department of Public Health; Center for Family Health; Maternal, Child, and Adolescent Health Division. The California Pregnancy-Associated Mortality Review (CA-PAMR) Report: pregnancy-associated suicide, 2002–2012. 2019. Available at: https://www.cmqcc.org/sites/default/files/PAMR%202.0%20Report_FINAL_8.8%20%281%29.pdf. Accessed January 15, 2023.
31. Ruhm CJ. Geographic variation in opioid and heroin involved drug poisoning mortality rates. *Am J Prev Med*. 2017;53(6):745–753. https://doi.org/10.1016/j.amepre.2017.06.009
32. Mertz KJ, Janssen JK, Williams KE. Underrepresentation of heroin involvement in unintentional drug overdose deaths in Allegheny County, PA. *J Forensic Sci*. 2014;59(6):1583–1585. https://doi.org/10.1111/1556-4029.12541
33. Trost S, Beauregard J, Njie F, Harvey A, Berry J, Goodman D. Pregnancy-related deaths among American Indian or Alaska Native persons: data from maternal mortality review committees in 36 US states, 2017–2019. Centers for Disease Control and Prevention. 2022. Available at: https://www.cdc.gov/reproductivehealth/maternal-mortality/erase-mm/data-mmrc.html. Accessed September 20, 2023.
34. Haffajee RL, Faherty LJ, Zivin K. Pregnant women with substance use disorders—the harm associated with punitive approaches. *N Engl J Med*. 2021;384(25):2364–2367. https://doi.org/10.1056/NEJMp2101051
35. Griffen A, McIntyre L, Belsito JZ, et al. Perinatal mental health care in the United States: an overview of policies and programs. *Health Aff (Millwood)*. 2021;40(10):1543–1550. https://doi.org/10.1377/hlthaff.2021.00796

Erratum In: "Characterizing the Burden of Occupational Chemical Exposures by Sociodemographic Groups in the United States, 2021"

In: Stephan-Recaido SC, Peckham TK, Lavoué Jerôme, Baker MG. Characterizing the burden of occupational chemical exposures by sociodemographic groups in the United States, 2021. *Am J Public Health*. 2024;114(1):57–67.

When originally published, the Figure and Table callouts were reported incorrectly. On p. 61, column 1, the first full paragraph should read:

Table 2 shows the estimated number and percentage of US workers exposed to the 10 most-prevalent chemical agents, stratified by sociodemographic group. Among all workers, the most-prevalent exposures were cleaning and antimicrobial agents (22.5 million US workers exposed; 14.7% of total workforce), engine emissions (19.5 million; 12.8%), organic solvents (18.5 million; 12.1%), polycyclic aromatic hydrocarbons (15.4 million; 10.1%), and diesel engine emissions (12.7 million; 8.3%). The prevalence of exposures varied across sociodemographic groups. Figure 1 shows the total number of exposures in which each sociodemographic group was disproportionately exposed. For both the 10 most prevalent agents and all agents combined, American Indian/Alaska Native, Hispanic/Latino, male, and foreign-born noncitizen workers; workers from REM groups as a whole; and workers with lower educational attainment were routinely overrepresented in exposure. Workers from other REM groups were estimated to experience disproportionate exposure to many of the 10 most-prevalent exposures, including Native Hawaiian/Pacific Islander (10 of 10), Black/African American (5 of 10), and multiracial (4 of 10) groups. Figure 2 shows the magnitude of overrepresentation of exposure to the 10 most-prevalent agents by sociodemographic group. Workers with lower educational attainment generally experienced increasingly greater magnitudes of disproportionate exposure, and Hispanic workers experienced the greatest magnitude of disproportionate exposure among all racial and ethnic groups.

The figures appeared out of order. On p. 61, Figure 1 should be:

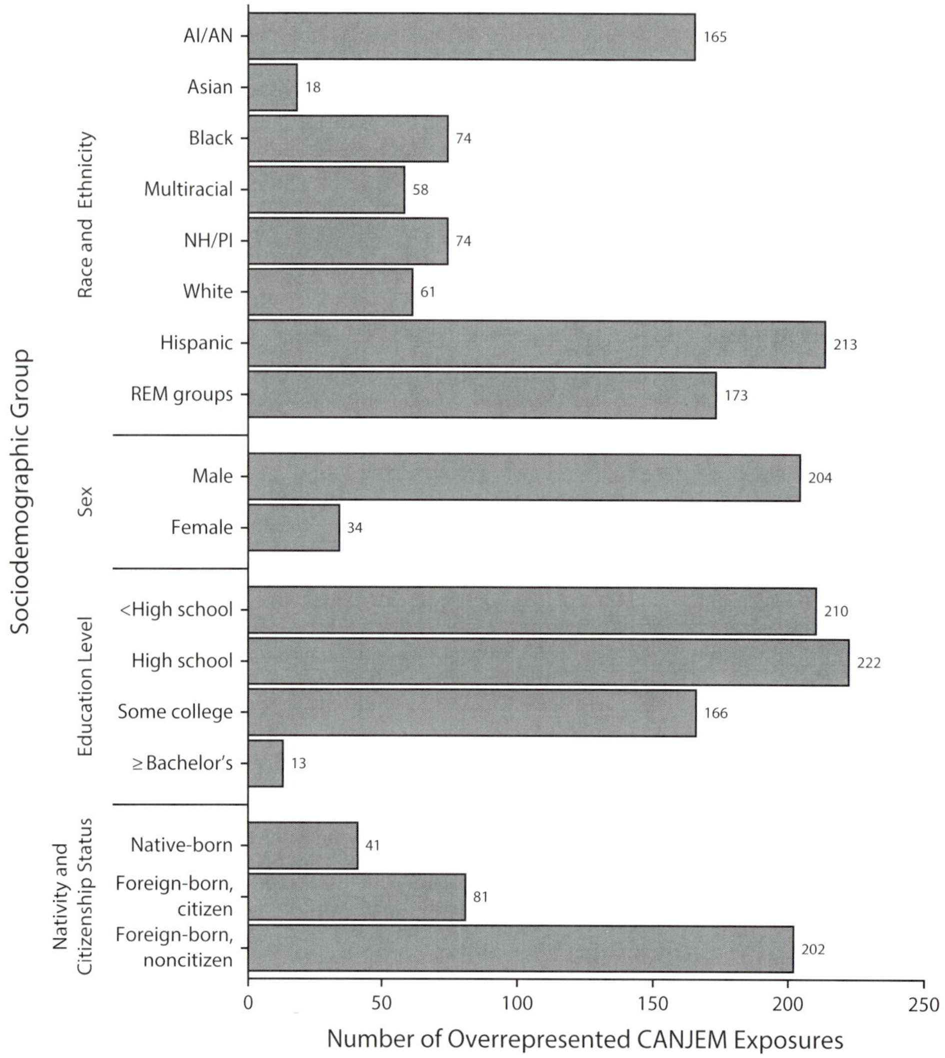

FIGURE 1— Total Number of Overrepresented Chemical CANJEM Exposures by Sociodemographic Group in the United States, 2021

Note. AI/AN = American Indian/Alaska Native; Black = Black/African American; CANJEM = Canadian job-exposure matrix; Hispanic = Hispanic/Latino; NH/PI = Native Hawaiian/Pacific Islander; REM groups = racial and ethnic minoritized groups; some college = some college or associate degree; White = non-Hispanic White. Persons within each race category are of any ethnicity, except for persons who identify as non-Hispanic White, and persons of Hispanic/Latino ethnicity are also counted in their preferred race category. REM groups include persons identifying as American Indian/Alaska Native, Asian, Black/African American, multiracial, Native Hawaiian/Pacific Islander, or Hispanic/Latino.

On p. 62, Figure 2 should be:

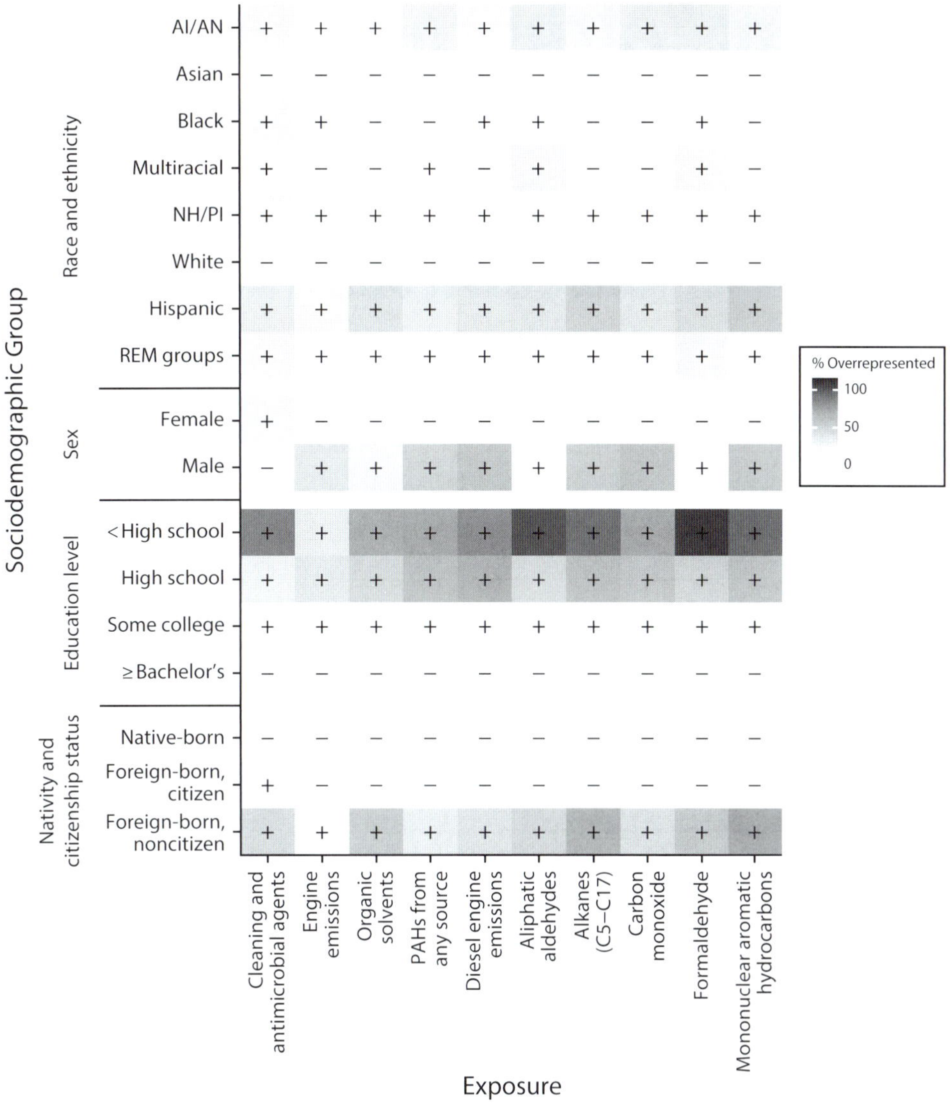

FIGURE 2— Magnitude of US Workers by Sociodemographic Group Overrepresented in Exposure to the 10 Most Prevalent Chemical Agents in CANJEM, 2021

Note. AI/AN = American Indian/Alaska Native; Black = Black/African American; CANJEM = Canadian job-exposure matrix; Hispanic = Hispanic/Latino; NH/PI = Native Hawaiian/Pacific Islander; PAHs = polycyclic aromatic hydrocarbons; REM groups = racial and ethnic minoritized groups; White = non-Hispanic White. A positive sign indicates overrepresentation of exposure (i.e., the number of workers exposed is in excess of the expected exposed based on the group's share of the total workforce). Darker shades of gray indicate higher percentages of overrepresentation. A negative sign indicates underrepresentation of exposure (i.e., the number of workers exposed is under the expected exposed based on the group's share of the total workforce). Persons within each race category are of any ethnicity, except for persons who identify as non-Hispanic White, and persons of Hispanic/Latino ethnicity are also counted in their preferred race category. REM groups include persons identifying as AI/AN, Asian, Black/African American, multiracial, Native Hawaiian/Pacific Islander, or Hispanic/Latino.

The article's full citation was listed incorrectly. On p. 66, the citation under the Publication Information section should read:

"Stephan-Recaido SC, Peckham TK, Lavoué J, Baker MG. Characterizing the burden of occupational chemical exposures by sociodemographic groups in the United States, 2021. *Am J Public Health*. 2024;114(1):57–67."

These changes do not affect the article's conclusions. AJPH

https://doi.org/10.2105/AJPH.2023.307461e

Erratum In: "Airborne Lead Exposure and Childhood Cognition: The Environmental Influences on Child Health Outcomes (ECHO) Cohort (2003–2022)"

In: Gatzke-Kopp LM, Willoughby M, Kress AM, et al. Airborne lead exposure and childhood cognition: the Environmental Influences on Child Health Outcomes (ECHO) cohort (2003–2022). *Am J Public Health*. 2024;114(3):309–318.

When originally published, the authorship order was listed incorrectly. On p. 309, the author byline should read:

Lisa M. Gatzke-Kopp, PhD, Michael Willoughby, PhD, Kristen McArthur, ScM, Cara Wychgram, MPP, David C. Folch, PhD, Steve Brunswasser, PhD, Dana Dabelea, MD, PhD, Amy J. Elliott, PhD, Tina Hartert, MD, MPH, Margaret Karagas, PhD, Cindy T. McEvoy, MD, MCR, James A. VanDerslice, PhD, Robert O. Wright, MD, MPH, Rosalind J. Wright, MD, and Amii M. Kress, PhD; on Behalf of Program Collaborators for Environmental Influences on Child Health Outcomes

On p. 317, the Publication Information section should read:

PUBLICATION INFORMATION

Full Citation: Gatzke-Kopp LM, Willoughby M, McArthur K, et al. Airborne lead exposure and childhood cognition: the Environmental Influences on Child Health Outcomes (ECHO) cohort (2003–2022). *Am J Public Health*. 2024;114(3):309–318.

Acceptance Date: October 27, 2023.

DOI: https://doi.org/10.2105/AJPH.2023.307519

ORCID iDs:

Lisa M. Gatzke-Kopp https://orcid.org/0000-0003-4470-4555

https://doi.org/10.2105/AJPH.2023.307519e

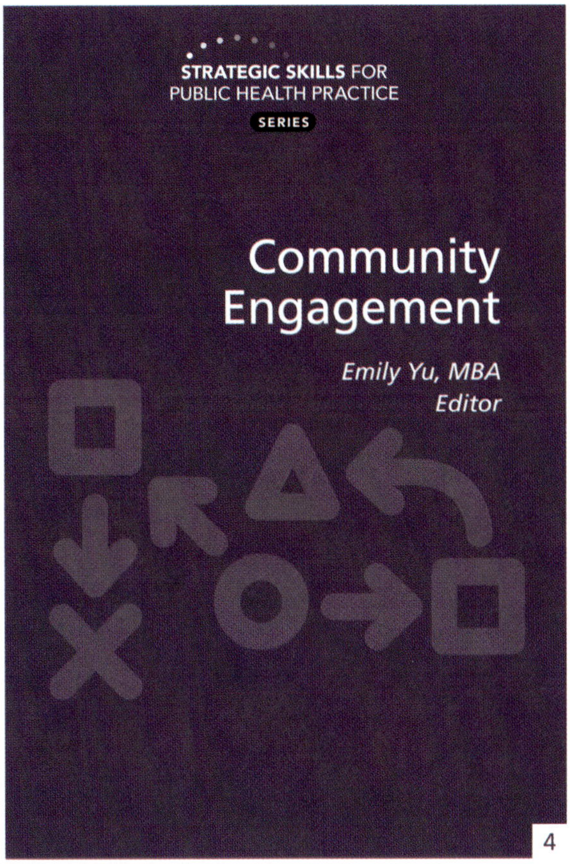

978-087553-3308, 108 PP, DIGITAL & SOFTCOVER

Community Engagement

Edited by Emily Yu, MBA

Community Engagement is the first book to be published from our new *Strategic Skills for Public Health Practice* series. This book brings the concept of community engagement to life through first-person stories, real-world examples and valuable insights from leaders across sectors. Curated specifically for public health practitioners and those interested in supporting community health, the book's chapters, guidance, and perspectives from the field will enhance readers' understanding of community-centered design and provide the tools to support organizational practices that drive better health for all.

APHABOOKSTORE.ORG

APHA PRESS

AN IMPRINT OF AMERICAN PUBLIC HEALTH ASSOCIATION

Standard Methods for the Examination of Dairy Products, 18th edition

Edited by Jeffrey L. Kornacki, PhD, Elliot T. Ryser, PhD, and Cynthia M. Mangione; Managing Editor: H. Michael Wehr, PhD

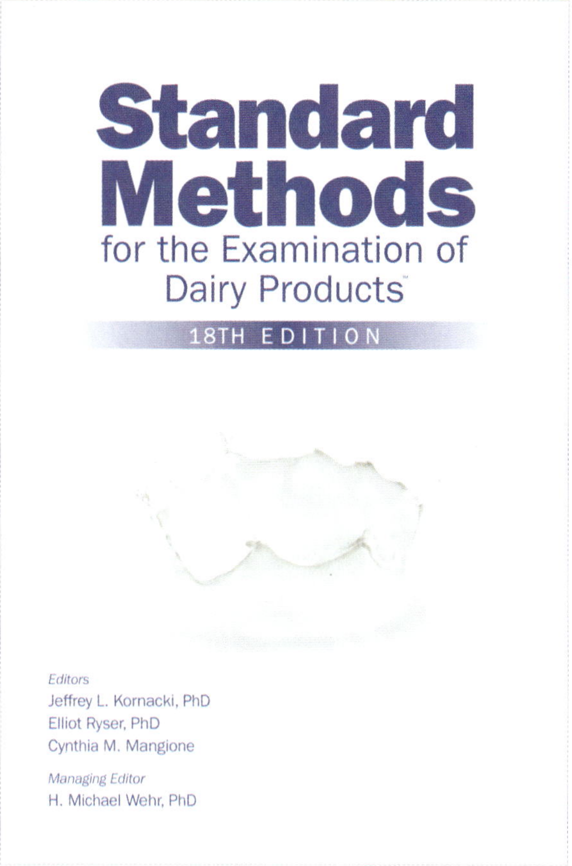

9780-887553-3421, SOFTCOVER, 1144 PP, 2024

Standard Methods for the Examination of Dairy Products is a widely-recognized source of methods to assess the safety and quality of dairy products. It is an overview of microbiological, chemical and physical methods for analyzing milk and dairy products, designed for use by regulatory, industry and commercial laboratories. As with earlier editions, the 18th edition of Standard Methods for the Examination of Dairy Products:

- Highlights test methods that are a critical component of both government and industry analytical programs.
- Provides methods that foster uniformity in the testing of milk and milk programs.

This new 18th Edition of SMEDP updates and expands upon earlier editions of this authoritative reference, including:

- Comprehensive revision to chapters on antibiotic drug residues, pathogens, chemical and physical methods, and methods for heat process verification.
- Updates on both automated, and molecular-based methods.

APHABOOKSTORE.ORG

APHA PRESS

AN IMPRINT OF AMERICAN PUBLIC HEALTH ASSOCIATION

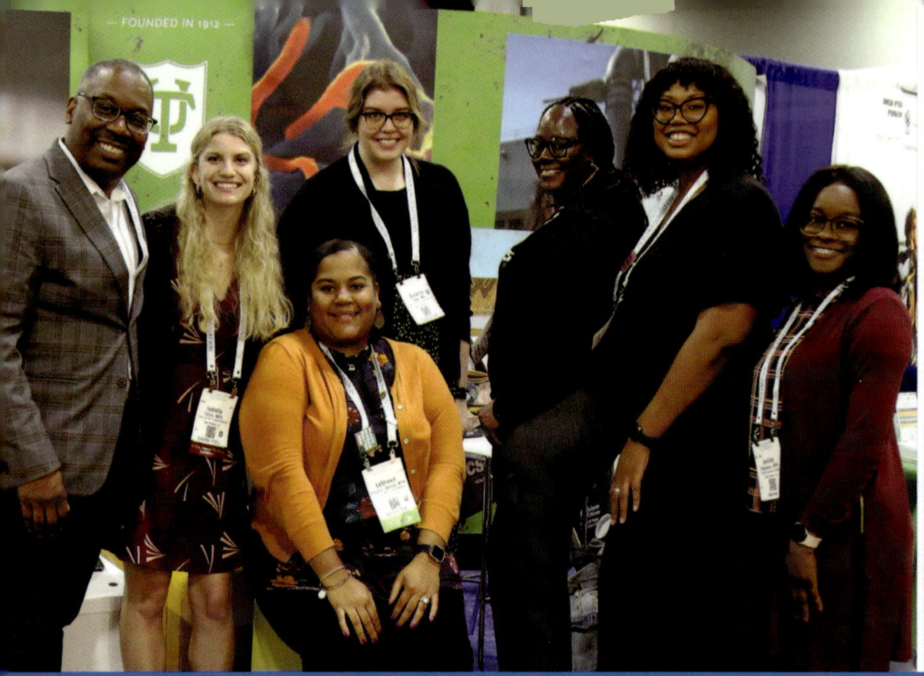
FOUNDED IN 1912
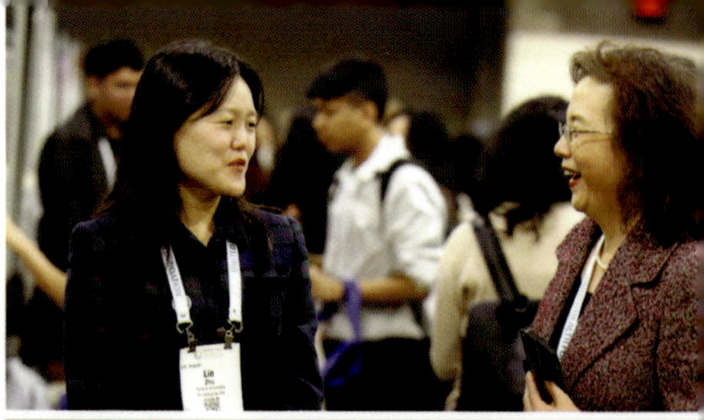
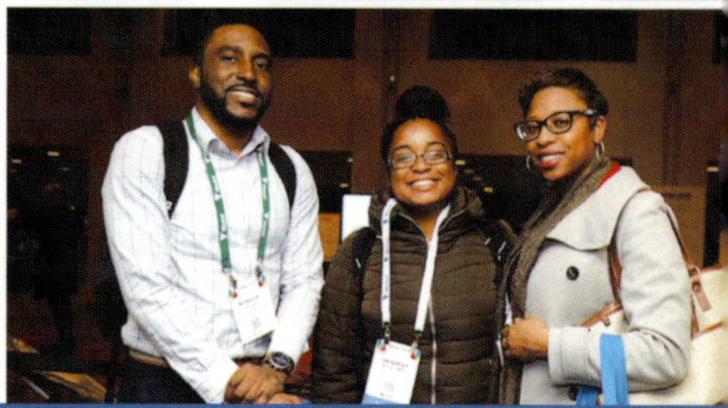